Objective Tests for Nurses
Book Three

Other books in the series contain questions on anatomy and physiology, and nursing care of medical and surgical conditions related to the following body systems:

Book One: The structure of the body

Book Two: The skeletal system and the muscular system

Forthcoming titles

Book Four: The digestive system and the urinary system

Book Five: The nervous system and the special senses

Book Six: The endocrine system and the female reproductive system

Objective Tests for Nurses
Book Three

The circulatory system and
the respiratory system

Compiled and edited by

Janet T. E. Riddle

RGN RFN ONC RNT(Edin)
Formerly Senior Tutor, College of Nursing and Midwifery,
Greater Glasgow Health Board, Western District

With contributions from

The late Joan Dinner

SRN RCNT
Formerly Clinical Teacher, Royal Hampshire County Hospital,
Winchester

May Lee

RGN SCM RCNT(Edin)
Clinical Nurse Teacher, Western District College of
Nursing and Midwifery, Glasgow

Rosa M. Sacharin

BA RSCN RGN SCM Dip N(Lond) RNT
Nurse Teacher, Western District College of Nursing
and Midwifery and Royal Hospital for Sick Children,
Yorkhill, Glasgow

Foreword by Margaret W. Thomson

RGN RSCN RNT SCM
Chief Executive Officer to the
National Board for Nursing, Midwifery
and Health Visiting for Scotland

CHURCHILL LIVINGSTONE
EDINBURGH LONDON MELBOURNE AND NEW YORK 1981

CHURCHILL LIVINGSTONE
Medical Division of Longman Group Limited

Distributed in the United States of America by
Churchill Livingstone Inc., 19 West 44th Street, New York,
N.Y. 10036, and by associated companies,
branches and representatives throughout
the world.

First published 1981

ISBN 0 443 01741 7

British Library Cataloguing in Publication Data

Riddle, Janet T. E.
    The circulatory system and the respiratory
    system—(Objective tests for nurses; book 3)
    1. Cardiovascular system—Diseases
    2. Cardiovascular disease nursing
    3. Respiratory organs—Diseases
    4. Respiratory disease nursing
    I. Title
    616.1'024613   RC667

Library of Congress Catalog Card Number
81–67468

Printed in Singapore by
Ban Wah Press

Foreword

The process of nursing has led nurses and nurse educators to be much more aware of the need to be objective in their approach to solving problems relating to nursing care given to patients. Since the first written examination for nurses, leading to registration with the General Council for Scotland, was held in 1925, the Council has endeavoured to construct a reliable means of ascertaining that candidates have reached a level of proficiency which will enable them to practise safely as Registered or Enrolled nurses.

The present system of examination consists of a written paper and a continuous assessment of proficiency in practice in the clinical areas: the former to test knowledge of facts and the understanding of the application of these facts to nursing practice, the latter to assess skills and attitudes which can more properly be assessed in a clinical setting.

The Council set up the Panel of Examiners which has given consideration to the format of the questions in the written paper and to the difficulties of their construction and marking relative to the various types.

The Council welcomed Churchill Livingstone's approach to assist in the compilation of a book which would be of interest to learners and assist them in their preparation to become Registered or Enrolled nurses. In order to encourage nurse teachers to participate in the compilation of the book, a workshop was sponsored by Churchill Livingstone under the auspices of the Department of Psychology at Moray House College of Education.

Although the General Nursing Council for Scotland has not so far included multiple choice questions in the final paper, the benefit to be gained from utilizing this book as a learning aid is to be commended. I trust that it will assist the learners to develop a questioning attitude and indeed provide some of the answers in order that they may become competent practitioners of nursing.

Margaret W. Thomson

About the series

Foreword

This series of books was devised in response to the ever-increasing demand for books which would give the nurse learner practice in answering objective tests. Each book in the series consists of questions on two body systems. Within each system the questions are split into (1) those on anatomy and physiology, and (2) those on case histories based on common disorders relating to each system.

However, the authors and publishers felt that in order to be really useful the books should be more than just a collection of questions and answers. We wanted the reader to be able to find out *why* one answer was considered right and another wrong and to understand the implications involved. For this reason the nursing care questions have been based on case histories and full explanatory answers are given in these sections.

Since we regarded the books as aids to learning and revision rather than as 'crammers' for examinations, we have not confined ourselves to the use of multiple choice questions only. Instead a variety of objective tests has been used and again it is hoped that this will make the books more interesting and useful to the reader.

The questions have been tested on different groups of nurse learners and all have been found to be appropriate. No attempt has been made to grade the questions; they have been written for the nurse learner who has completed the first eighteen months of training. All the results have been evaluated by computer and subsequently analysed and any questions of doubtful ambiguity have been omitted.

Finally we felt it to be most important that the page layout used should provide space for the reader to make individual notes against the questions. For this reason we have used a page size considerably larger than is usual in books of this type.

We would emphasize that the book should be used in conjunction with other texts. A pre-knowledge of anatomy and physiology has been assumed and for further reference the reader is referred to the books in the short bibliography all of which are published by Churchill Livingstone.

Bibliography

Bloom: *Toohey's Medicine for Nurses*
Moroney: *Surgery for Nurses*
Riddle: *Anatomy and Physiology Applied to Nursing*
Ross and Wilson: *Foundations of Anatomy and Physiology*
Chilman and Thomas: *Understanding Nursing Care*

Preface

Many nurse teachers have experimented for a number of years with different types of objective test questions. This form of examination paper is becoming more popular and there is a need to produce questions for student and pupil nurses to use for practice and revision. Most of the books of this type are geared to the needs of medical students or are American publications couched in unfamiliar terminology so an attempt has been made to produce a series suitable for British nurses.

Although the main part of this book deals with nursing, some anatomy and physiology questions have been included. These are very basic and are aimed at testing the student's previous knowledge of the subject. The questions should be studied with a textbook on hand for reference, revision and further study.

In the nursing studies the authors have attempted to cover many aspects of nursing care and to form questions which test knowledge of facts, principles, understanding and evaluation. Each case study is followed by explanations, in some detail, of why the correct answer was selected. The student may not always agree with the answer, but it should be remembered that this book is not an examination and the authors will be pleased if it stimulates further study and discussion.

As editor, I would like to take this opportunity of thanking all the contributors who, after the sad and untimely death of Miss Joan Dinner, are helping to complete the series. We have attempted to continue with the format as first envisaged by Miss Dinner and we hope that the series will continue to reflect not only her inspiration but the tremendous amount of work she put into the first two volumes.

I would like to express my gratitude to Mrs Mary Law of Churchill Livingstone who has not only helped with the editing but has spent a great deal of time having the questions tested and evaluated. Her enthusiasm has inspired us all.

I would like to thank the nurses who took the tests and the tutors who administered them. Also the members of the staff of the computer centre at Moray House College of Education who produced the results and evaluations. My thanks also go to Miss J Ross and Dr K Wilson for allowing us to use some of their illustrations and to many friends who have given help and encouragement.

1981   Janet T. E. Riddle

Preface

Contents

Anatomy and physiology of the blood, circulation and respiration

Matching item questions

The following questions (1–21) are all of the matching item type. They consist of two lists. On the left is a list of lettered items (A, B, C etc.). On the right is a list of numbered items. Study the two lists and for each item in the numbered list select the appropriate item from the lettered list. You may indicate your answer by writing the appropriate letter in the right-hand margin.

Note. There are more items in the lettered list than in the numbered lists and you will therefore not use all the items in the lettered list. The answers to these questions may be found on page 17.

Cardiovascular system

1–3. From the list on the left select the tissue which forms each part of the wall of the heart listed on the right.

A. Areolar tissue   1. Endocardium   1.
B. Cardiac muscle tissue
C. Fibrous tissue   2. Myocardium   2.
D. Squamous epithelium
E. Voluntary muscle tissue   3. Pericardium   3.

4–6. From the list on the left select the tissue which forms each part of the wall of the arteries on the right.

A. Areolar tissue   4. Tunica adventitia   4.
B. Cardiac muscle tissue
C. Fibrous tissue   5. Tunica intima   5.
D. Involuntary muscle tissue
E. Squamous epithelium   6. Tunica media   6.

7–9. From the list on the left select the vessels which enter or leave the chambers of the heart listed on the right.

A. Aorta   7. Right atrium   7.
B. Superior vena cava
C. Coronary artery   8. Left atrium   8.
D. Pulmonary veins
E. Pulmonary artery   9. Left ventricle   9.

10–12. From the list on the left select the blood supply for the organs listed on the right.

A. Carotid   10. Bowel   10.
B. Gastric
C. Hepatic   11. Brain   11.
D. Mesenteric
E. Renal   12. Liver   12.

13–15. From the list on the left select the substance, present in plasma, which is best described by each word on the right.

A. Albumin

B. Enzyme

C. Glycerol

D. Potassium

E. Urea

13. Mineral   13.

14. Protein   14.

15. Waste   15.

Respiratory system

16–18. From the list on the left select the part of the nose formed by each bone listed on the right.

A. Anterior wall

B. Floor

C. Posterior wall

D. Roof

E. Septum

16. Nasal bones   16.

17. Palatine bones   17.

18. Vomer   18.

19–21. From the list on the left select the gas present in expired air in the percentage volume listed on the right.

A. Carbon dioxide

B. Inert gas

C. Nitrogen

D. Oxygen

E. Water vapour

19. 17%   19.

20. 4.04%   20.

21. 1%   21.

Multiple choice questions

The following questions (22–44) are all of multiple choice type. Read the questions and from the four possible answers select the ONE which you think is correct. You may indicate your answer by writing the appropriate letter in the right-hand margin. The answers to these questions may be found on page 17.

Cardiovascular system

22. The total blood volume in an adult is approximately:
    A. 2 litres
    B. 5 litres
    C. 8 litres
    D. 10 litres.

    22.

23. The blood is:
    A. Strongly acid
    B. Slightly acid
    C. Neutral
    D. Slightly alkaline.

    23.

24. The red blood corpuscles are:
    A. Erythrocytes
    B. Leucocytes
    C. Lymphocytes
    D. Thrombocytes.

    24.

25. Which one of the following constituents of blood plasma is necessary for the clotting of blood?
    A. Albumin
    B. Amino acids
    C. Creatinine
    D. Fibrinogen.

    25.

26. Bile pigment is a product of the break-down of:
    A. Erythrocytes
    B. Leucocytes
    C. Lymphocytes
    D. Thrombocytes.

    26.

27. Which one of the following statements is true? The blood travels from:
    A. The left atrium to the aorta
    B. The left ventricle to the vena cava
    C. The right ventricle to the pulmonary artery
    D. The right atrium to the pulmonary veins.

    27.

28. Which one of the following will slow the rate of the heart?   28.
    A. Emotion
    B. Exercise
    C. Haemorrhage
    D. Physical training.

29. The Cardiac cycle normally occurs: 29.
    A. Once in 1 second
    B. Once in 0.1 second
    C. Once in 0.3 second
    D. Once in 0.8 second

30. Arteries are lined with: 30.
    A. Epithelial tissue
    B. Fibrous tissue
    C. Lymphoid tissue
    D. Muscle tissue

31. The veins have valves, the function of which is to: 31.
    A. Maintain the flow of blood from the heart to the periphery
    B. Maintain the flow of blood to the heart
    C. Prevent the back flow of blood to the limbs
    D. Prevent the onward flow of blood from the capillaries.

32. Which one of the following is part of the blood supply to the brain?   32.
    A. Facial artery
    B. Internal carotid artery
    C. Left subclavian artery
    D. Temporal artery.

33. Which one of the following statements is true?   33.
    A. Lymphatic capillaries are less permeable than blood capillaries
    B. Lymphatic ducts enter the subclavian arteries.
    C. Lymphatic nodes are similar to glands with ducts
    D. Lymphatic vessels contain valves.

34. In which one of the following regions of the abdomen does the spleen lie?   34.
    A. Epigastric
    B. Hypogastric
    C. Left hypochondriac
    D. Right iliac.

Respiratory system

35. The interchange of gases takes place in:
    A. The air sacs
    B. The bronchi
    C. The nose
    D. The trachea.

36. Which of the following organs belongs to both the respiratory and digestive systems?
    A. Bronchi
    B. Larynx
    C. Oesophagus
    D. Pharynx.

37. The nasal cavity is lined with:
    A. Ciliated epithelium
    B. Cuboid epithelium
    C. Simple epithelium
    D. Squamous epithelium.

38. The vocal cords are situated in the:
    A. Larynx
    B. Lungs
    C. Pharynx
    D. Trachea.

39. The tissue joining the lobules of the lungs is:
    A. Cartilage
    B. Elastic tissue
    C. Epithelial tissue
    D. Muscle tissue.

40. Which one of the following statements is true? The pleura is:
    A. A fibrous membrane
    B. A mucous membrane
    C. A serous membrane
    D. A synovial membrane.

41. Which one of the following statements is true? The parietal layer of the pleura:
    A. Covers the diaphragm
    B. Covers the thoracic vertebrae
    C. Covers the lungs
    D. Covers the bronchi.

35.

36.

37.

38.

39.

40.

41.

42. The auditory tubes (pharyngo-tympanic) carry air:
    A. From the air sinuses to the ear
    B. From the nasopharynx to the middle ear
    C. From the nose to the inner ear
    D. From the oropharynx to the outer ear.

42.

43. During expiration:
    A. The air sacs empty completely
    B. The diaphragm flattens
    C. The intercostal muscles contract
    D. The lungs recoil.

43.

44. Inspired air contains:
    A. Oxygen—78%
    B. Nitrogen—21%
    C. Carbon dioxide—0.04%
    D. Argon—3%.

44.

Matching item questions using a diagram

The following questions (45–80) all consist of a diagram with numbered parts. With each diagram there is a list of named parts (A, B, C etc.). Look at the diagram and for each numbered structure select a name from the list of parts. You may indicate your answer by writing the appropriate letter in the right-hand margin. Answers may be found on page 17.

Note. There are more lettered items than numbers on the diagram so you will not use all the names in the lists.

Cardiovascular system

45–47. Blood cells
    A. Erythrocyte
    B. Leucocyte
    C. Thrombocytes

45.
46.
47.

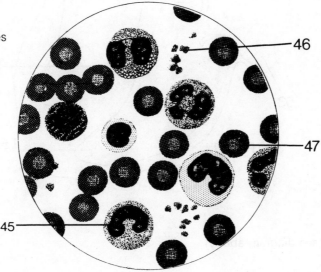

48–50. The heart

    A. Aortic valve
    B. Bicuspid valve
    C. Pulmonary valve
    D. Pulmonary vein
    E. Tricuspid valve

48.

49.

50.

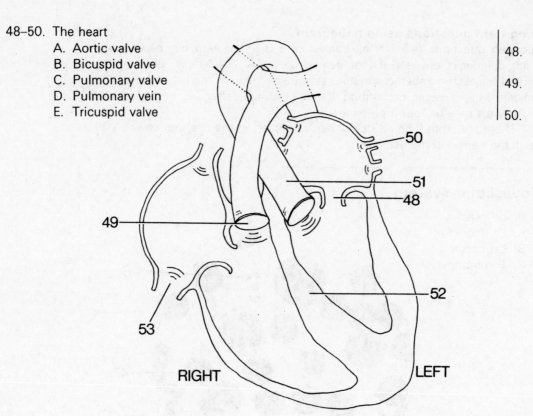

RIGHT   LEFT

51–53. The heart (see diagram above)

    A. Aorta
    B. Endocardium
    C. Pulmonary artery
    D. Septum
    E. Vena cava

51.

52.

53.

54–56. The arterial blood supply
    A. Axillary
    B. Common carotid
    C. Radial
    D. Subclavian
    E. Ulnar

54.

55.

56.

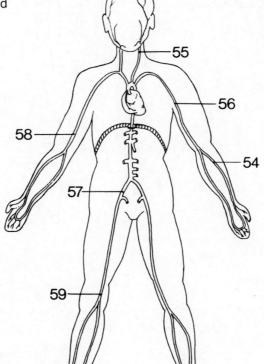

57–59. The arterial blood supply (see diagram above)
    A. Aorta
    B. Brachial
    C. Common iliac
    D. Femoral
    E. Popliteal.

57.

58.

59.

60–62. The arch of the aorta and the superior vena cava
    A. Axillary vein
    B. Common carotid artery
    C. Jugular vein
    D. Pulmonary vein
    E. Subclavian vein.

60.

61.

62.

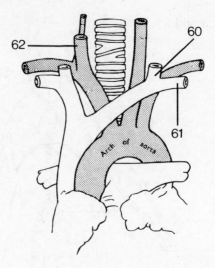

63–65. Veins and lymphatics
    A. Jugular vein
    B. Mediastinal nodes
    C. Occipital nodes
    D. Plantar vein
    E. Thoracic duct.

63.

64.

65.

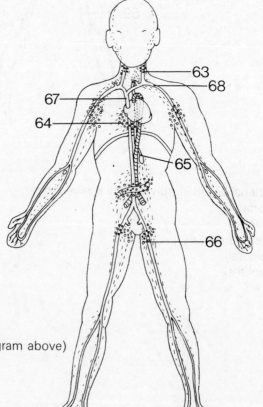

66–68. Veins and lymphatics (see diagram above)
    A. Axillary nodes
    B. Inguinal nodes
    C. Popliteal vein
    D. Subclavian vein
    E. Superior vena cava.

66.

67.

68.

Respiratory system

69–71. The respiratory system
  A. Bronchus
  B. Pharynx
  C. Pleura
  D. Thyroid cartilage
  E. Trachea.

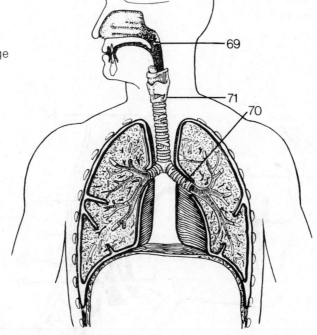

69.

70.

71.

72–74. An air sac
  A. Alveolus
  B. Branch of the pulmonary artery
  C. Branch of the pulmonary vein
  D. Bronchiole

72.

73.

74.

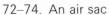
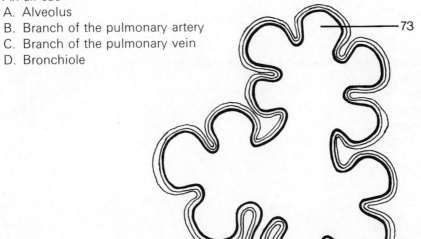

Venous blood   Arterial blood

75–77. Section through head and neck
   A. Adenoids
   B. Hyoid bone
   C. Oropharynx
   D. Uvula.

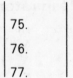

75.

76.

77.

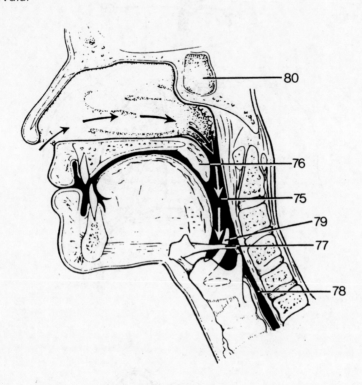

78–80. Section through head and neck (see diagram above)
   A. Cricoid cartilage
   B. Epiglottis
   C. Nasal sinus
   D. Oesophagus
   E. Thyroid cartilage.

78.

79.

80.

True/false questions

The following questions (81–184) consist of a number of statements, some of which are true and some of which are false. Consider each statement and decide whether you think it is true or false. You can indicate your answer by writing T for true or F for false in the right-hand margin beside each statement. Answers may be found on page 17.

81–84. Erthrocytes:
    81. Produce Vitamin B   81.
    82. Protect against infection   82.
    83. Synthesize haemoglobin   83.
    84. Transport oxygen.   84.

85–88. Haemoglobin:
    85. Contains iron   85.
    86. Is a carbohydrate   86.
    87. Requires cyancobalamine (Vitamin B_{12})   87.
    88. Transports oxygen.   88.

89–92. Leucocytes:
    89. Are concerned with immunity   89.
    90. Are motile   90.
    91. Ingest bacteria   91.
    92. Produce thrombin.   92.

93–96. In normal blood the number of:
    93. Erythrocytes exceeds the number of leucocytes   93.
    94. Erythrocytes is greater in women than in men   94.
    95. Leucocytes is greater than the number of thrombocytes   95.
    96. Thrombocytes is less than the number of erythrocytes.   96.

97–100. The plasma:
    97. Contains calcium   97.
    98. Contains haemoglobin   98.
    99. Is the other name for serum   99.
    100. Is about 90% water.   100.

101–104. When a transfusion of blood is necessary a person who belongs to group:
    101. A can give blood to group O   101.
    102. AB can receive blood from group A   102.
    103. B can receive blood from group AB   103.
    104. O can give blood to group O.   104.

105–108. The heart lies:
    105. Above the diaphragm   105.
    106. Between the lungs   106.
    107. Behind the thoracic aorta   107.
    108. In front of the oesophagus.   108.

109–112. The endocardium:
    109. Forms the valves of the heart   109.
    110. Is continuous with the lining of the blood vessels   110.
    111. Is made of epithelium   111.
    112. Is a serous membrane.   112.

113–116. The myocardium:
    113. Forms the septum of the heart   113.
    114. Is a continuation of the muscular wall of the arteries   114.
    115. Is the muscular wall of the heart   115.
    116. Is thicker at the base of the heart than the apex.   116.

117–120. The pericardium:
    117. Controls the heart beat   117.
    118. Controls the flow of blood   118.
    119. Prevents over-distension of the heart   119.
    120. Prevents friction.   120.

121–124. When the skin arterioles constrict:
    121. Heat is lost from the body   121.
    122. The blood pressure rises   122.
    123. The pulse rate increases   123.
    124. The skin becomes pale.   124.

125–128. The blood capillaries are:
    125. Formed by branches of the veins   125.
    126. Found in all organs   126.
    127. Made of fibrous tissue   127.
    128. Semipermeable   128.

129–132. Osmotic pressure is the force which:
    129. Draws tissue fluid through the walls of the capillaries   129.
    130. Pushes the fluid from the blood to the tissue cells   130.
    131. Returns the blood to the heart   131.
    132. Sends the blood into the general circulation.   132.

133–136. The veins
    133. The brachial vein is a continuation of the axillary vein   133.
    134. The gastric vein enters the inferior vena cava   134.
    135. The hepatic veins are branches of the portal vein   135.
    136. The jugular veins join the subclavian veins.   136.

137–140. Blood pressure is:
    137. Decreased by standing still   137.
    138. Decreased by the application of cold   138.
    139. Increased in shock   139.
    140. Increased in emotion.   140.

141–144. Diastole and systole are part of the cardiac cycle. During diastole:
    141. The atria and ventricles are relaxed   141.
    142. The atrial and ventricular valves are closed   142.
    143. The blood is entering the heart by the pulmonary veins   143.
    144. The blood pressure is increased.   144.

145–148. During systole:
    145. The aortic valve closes   145.
    146. Blood is pushed into the pulmonary artery.   146.
    147. The blood pressure in an adult is usually about 120 mm Hg   147.
    148. The ventricles contract before the atria.   148.

149–152. In the lymphatic system:
    149. The right duct drains the right side of the abdomen   149.
    150. The right duct enters the right subclavian artery   150.
    151. The thoracic duct receives lymph from both legs.   151.
    152. The lymphatic vessels of the abdomen enter the thoracic duct   152.
        above the diaphragm.

153–156. The spleen forms:
    153. Antibodies   153.
    154. Antitoxins   154.
    155. Lymphocytes   155.
    156. Erythrocytes.   156.

157–160. Antibodies:
      157. Are always acquired naturally
      158. Are destroyed by thrombocytes
      159. Are produced by lymphocytes
      160. Respond to any type of infection.

157.
158.
159.
160.

Respiratory system

161–164. The pharynx:
      161. Contains the adenoids
      162. Is continuous with the oesophagus
      163. Is made of cartilage
      164. Lies in front of the thoracic vertebrae.

161.
162.
163.
164.

165–168 In the larynx:
      165. The cricoid cartilage is attached to the trachea
      166. The epiglottis is attached to the cricoid cartilage
      167. The thyroid cartilage is attached to the hyoid bone
      168. The vocal cords are attached to the thyroid cartilage.

165.
166.
167.
168.

169–172. The trachea:
      169. Is composed of incomplete rings of cartilage
      170. Is continuous with the pharynx
      171. Divides to form the bronchioles
      172. Is lined with ciliated mucous membrane.

169.
170.
171.
172.

173–176. The bronchi:
      They lie behind the oesophagus
      They lie in front of the heart
      175. The left bronchus is longer than the right
      176. The right bronchus divides into three branches.

173.
174.
175.
176.

177–180. The bronchioles:
      177. Are continuous with the air sacs
      178. Are lined with ciliated columnar epithelium
      179. Have cartilage in their walls
      180. Have a diameter of one centimetre.

177.
178.
179.
180.

181–184. During inspiration:
      181. The chest wall falls
      182. The chest wall rises
      183. The diaphragm falls
      184. The diaphragm rises.

181.
182.
183.
184.

Answers (Questions 1 to 184)

Matching items *(Page 1)*

1. D	7. B	13. D	19. D
2. B	8. D	14. A	20. A
3. C	9. A	15. E	21. B
4. C	10. D	16. A	
5. E	11. A	17. B	
6. D	12. C	18. E	

Multiple choice *(Page 3)*

22. B	28. D	34. C	40. C
23. D	29. D	35. A	41. A
24. A	30. A	36. D	42. B
25. D	31. C	37. A	43. D
26. A	32. B	38. A	44. C
27. C	33. D	39. B	

Matching items using a diagram *(Page 7)*

45. B	54. C	63. A	72. B
46. C	55. B	64. B	73. A
47. A	56. A	65. E	74. D
48. B	57. C	66. B	75. C
49. C	58. B	67. E	76. D
50. D	59. E	68. D	77. B
51. A	60. C	69. B	78. D
52. D	61. E	70. A	79. B
53. E	62. B	71. D	80. C

True/false *(Page 13)*

81. False	93. True	105. True	117. False
82. False	94. False	106. True	118. False
83. True	95. False	107. False	119. True
84. True	96. True	108. True	120. True
85. True	97. True	109. True	121. False
86. False	98. False	110. True	122. True
87. True	99. False	111. True	123. False
88. True	100. True	112. False	124. True
89. True	101. False	113. True	125. False
90. True	102. True	114. False	126. True
91. True	103. False	115. True	127. False
92. False	104. True	116. False	128. True

129. True	143. True	157. False	171. False
130. False	144. False	158. False	172. True
131. False	145. False	159. True	173. False
132. False	146. True	160. False	174. False
133. True	147. True	161. True	175. True
134. False	148. False	162. True	176. True
135. False	149. False	163. False	177. True
136. True	150. False	164. False	178. True
137. True	151. True	165. True	179. False
138. False	152. False	166. False	180. False
139. False	153. True	167. True	181. False
140. True	154. True	168. True	182. True
141. True	155. True	169. True	183. True
142. False	156. False	170. False	184. False

Acute juvenile rheumatism (rheumatic fever)

The following questions (185–264) are based on the case history given below.

James is 10 years old. He has been admitted to the hospital because of recurrent fleeting pains in various joints. He is one of three children. His birth was normal and there is no family history of heart disease. He has had an uneventful sickness record but had chickenpox and measles without any complications.

All the children have had recent throat infections and although James had been confined to bed for a few days he responded readily to antibiotic treatment. He returned to school a week later. James was an active child but his mother noticed that he tended recently to sit around much more and in fact seemed quite lethargic. His appetite was not as good as it had been and he was rather pale. His temperature was normal, but he complained of some pain in his knees, arms and shoulders. On the day of admission to hospital, he did not want to get up, was weepy and complained of abdominal pain. His general practitioner was called, and decided to have him admitted to hospital. James arrived in the ward on a trolley. The provisional diagnosis was 'acute juvenile rheumatism'.

Multiple choice questions

The following questions (185–220) are all of the multiple choice type. Read the questions and from the possible answers select the ONE which you think is correct. You may indicate your answer by writing the appropriate letter against the number in the right-hand margin.

185. Which of the following should the nurse ascertain first?   185.
    A. His general condition
    B. His level of anxiety
    C. Time of his last meal
    D. Parents' reaction to his admission.

186. When deciding on the best way to admit James, the nurse should assess: 186.
    A. The amount of pain present
    B. His attitude towards admission
    C. His ability to walk
    D. His state of cleanliness.

187. On the basis of your assessment, which of the following items of equipment   187.
would be most useful for James?
    A. Additional blankets
    B. A bedcage
    C. Side rails
    D. Additional pillows.

188. Which of the following would you consider should be done first?   188.
    A. Take his temperature, pulse and respirations
    B. Take his blood pressure
    C. Weigh him
    D. Bath him.

189. James complains of moderate pain, particularly in his knees and elbows.   189.
Which of the following methods would you use for bathing him?
    A. Shower
    B. Bedbath
    C. Ordinary bath
    D. Allow him to wash himself.

190. On admission children are weighed and measured. Which of the following   190.
describes the reason most accurately?
    A. To assess normal development
    B. To assess weight gain
    C. As a criterion for calculating drug dosage
    D. For research purposes.

191. In order to obtain a picture of James' personality and to provide a suitable   191.
nursing care plan the nurse should obtain information about him from one
of the following:
    A. Teacher
    B. Doctor
    C. Parents
    D. Form her own opinion.

192. What other type of information should the nurse obtain to help her provide   192.
the right environment for James?
    A. Relationship with other children
    B. Likes and dislikes
    C. Any contact with an infectious disease
    D. All of the above.

To establish the diagnosis and to determine involvement of various organs, a number of investigations and tests will be necessary. Some of these are nursing functions, others involve the doctor with assistance from the nurse.

193. Since James has had a history of recurrent throat infection, a throat swab will be taken. Which of the following areas will provide the best specimen?
    A. Tonsillar region and tongue
    B. Tongue and buccal mucosa
    C. Uvula and tongue
    D. Tonsillar region and nose.

194. So that the least discomfort is caused to the child, the following steps should be taken by the nurse. Which one is *not* essential?
    A. Explain the procedure and gain his co-operation
    B. Hold his head firmly
    C. Have him lying flat
    D. Hold his hands to prevent him handling the swab.

195. In order to obtain a successful swab, the nurse should:
    A. Gently touch the tonsillar region with the swab-stick
    B. Gently and quickly draw the swab-stick across the tonsillar region
    C. Take time to swab the area
    D. Make sure that all exudate has been removed from the tonsils.

196. The swab will be sent to which of the following departments?
    A. Biochemistry
    B. Pathology
    C. Bacteriology
    D. Oncology.

197. The swabs will be tested to determine:
    A. The identity of organisms present
    B. Sensitivity to antibodies
    C. The number of colonies present
    D. All of the above.

198. Which of the following organisms most commonly causes throat infection?
    A. Streptococcus viridans
    B. Staphylococcus aureus
    C. B-Haemolytic streptococcus
    D. Diplococcus.

193.

194.

195.

196.

197

198.

199. James looks pale, it is therefore necessary to analyse his: 199.
    A. Urine for presence of blood
    B. Faecal occult blood
    C. Blood
    D. Plasma.

200. Which of the following tests should be carried out to aid diagnosis?   200.
    A. Erythrocyte sedimentation rate
    B. X-ray of chest
    C. Electrocardiogram
    D. All of the above.

201. In acute juvenile rheumatism one would expect the erythrocyte
    sedimentation rate to be: 201.
    A. Increased
    B. Normal
    C. Decreased
    D. Fluctuating.

James complains of joint pains. He is lethargic and anorexic.

---

202. Which of the following drugs is most likely to be prescribed to give James   202.
    relief from pain?
    A. Indomethacin
    B. Codeine
    C. Aspirin
    D. Paracetamol.

203. Which of the following drugs is most likely to be prescribed to help protect   203.
    James from recurrent B-haemolytic streptococcal infection?
    A. Sulphadiazine
    B. Streptomycin
    C. Penicillin
    D. Neomycin.

204. When giving salicylates which of the following signs indicate toxicity?   204.
    A. Overbreathing
    B. Tinnitus and deafness
    C. Nausea and vomiting
    D. All of the above.

205. Before giving penicillin it is necessary to determine:
     A. The type of penicillin previously given, if any
     B. That he is not allergic to penicillin
     C. That the organism is sensitive to penicillin
     D. That kidney function is normal.

     205.

206. Which of the following signs indicate an allergic reaction?
     A. Increased body temperature
     B. Skin rash
     C. Swelling of the face, throat and joints
     D. All of the above.

     206.

James has been on salicylates for a week but there has not been the dramatic improvement usually expected. There is also evidence of carditis. The doctor prescribes adrenocortical steroids.

---

207. Which of the following are likely effects of steroid therapy?
     A. Moon face
     B. Arrest of growth
     C. Increased susceptibility to infection
     D. All of the above.

     207.

208. During the acute phase of the condition the child should be:
     A. Kept on complete bed rest
     B. Allowed limited mobility
     C. Allowed up in the afternoon
     D. Allowed up to the toilet.

     208.

209. Which of the following observations should be made to monitor progress?
     A. 2-hourly temperature, pulse and respiration and hourly blood pressure
     B. 2-hourly temperature, pulse and respiration and sleeping pulse
     C. 4-hourly temperature, pulse and respiration and daily blood pressure
     D. 4-hourly temperature, pulse and respiration and sleeping pulse.

     209.

210. In view of the fact that James' joints are painful and he is reluctant to move, which of the following nursing measures would be important in preventing skin damage?
     A. Frequent turning
     B. Ripple bed
     C. Encourage limited movements
     D. All of the above.

     210.

211. James' appetite is poor. Which of the following diets would you consider   211.
     most suitable during the *acute* phase?
     A. Fluid
     B. Soft
     C. High protein
     D. Normal.

212. A chart is kept to record James' fluid intake and output. It is important that   212.
     this is accurately maintained to ensure that:
     A. The child receives drinks at regular intervals
     B. The child is not dehydrated
     C. The kidneys are functioning properly
     D. He is receiving adequate nutrients.

213. James is not keen to take aspirin tablets because he feels nauseated. Which   213.
     of the following methods might help him to accept and retain the tablets?
     A. Crushing the tablets
     B. Changing the analgesic
     C. Giving a smaller dosage
     D. Giving soluble aspirin tablets.

214. Which of the following describes a heart murmur?   214.
     A. The noise caused by the opening of a heart valve
     B. The noise caused by the flow of blood through a valve
     C. The noise heard over areas of the cardiovascular system where blood
        flow is turbulent
     D. The noise heard over areas of the cardiovascular system where blood
        vessels are narrowed.

215. When nursing a child with acute juvenile rheumatism it is important to   215.
     recognize early signs of complications. Which of the following indicates
     early cardiac involvement?
     A. A decrease in pulse rate during rest
     B. An increase in pulse rate during activity
     C. A persistently high sleeping pulse rate
     D. An irregular pulse rate.

216. Which part of the heart is *least* likely to be affected?   216.
     A. Endocardium
     B. Pericardium
     C. Myocardium
     D. Mitral valve.

217. James is given steroids (prednisone). This drug may cause obesity. Which
of the following dietary measures can be taken to prevent this?
A. High roughage
B. Low calorie
C. Low carbohydrates and low sodium
D. Low protein and low carbohydrate.

217.

Following the administration of prednisone there is an improvement
in James' general condition. His ESR is normal and his sleeping
pulse rate is within normal limits.

---

218. Which of the following rates of sleeping pulse could be considered within
normal limits for a boy of 10?
A. 70–80 beats per minute
B. 90–106 beats per minute
C. 86–96 beats per minute
D. 68–76 beats per minute.

218.

219. The doctor considers that James can be allowed up. What decision would
you make regarding his period of activity?
A. Allow him up for gradually increasing periods
B. Allow him up for the same time as the other active children
C. Allow him up till he shows signs of tiredness
D. Tell him to let you know when he wants to return to bed.

219.

220. Which of the following observations should the nurse make while James
is up?
A. Colour
B. Breathing rate
C. Pulse rate and rhythm
D. Temperature.

220.

His improvement is maintained and the prednisone and aspirin are being discontinued gradually. James is now ready to go home.

True/false questions

The following questions (221–228) consist of a number of statements, some of which are true and some of which are false. Consider each statement and decide whether you think it is true or false. You can indicate your answer by writing T for true or F for false in the right-hand margin beside each statement.

What advice would the parents be given?

221. James should continue taking penicillin until he is 18 years old.   221.

222. He should gradually increase his activities.   222.

223. There should be no restrictions on his activity.   223.

224. He can go back to school as soon as he is discharged.   224.

225. His diet should be restricted.   225.

226. He should remain isolated for at least four weeks to avoid becoming infected by others.   226.

227. He should attend the out-patient department at regular intervals.   227.

228. He should be given penicillin and streptomycin whenever major dental work is necessary.   228.

Following his discharge from hospital, James was able to return to school. The remainder of his childhood passed normally and he did not have any further periods of illness. However, as a result of his attack of carditis he was left with residual heart disease. This did not bother him until he was middle-aged, when he suffered an attack of bacterial endocarditis.

Multiple choice questions
The following questions (229–235) are of the multiple choice type. Read the questions and from the possible answers select the ONE which you think is correct.

229. Which of the following structures is *most* likely to be affected by damage from bacterial endocarditis?
    A. Aortic valve
    B. Mitral valve
    C. Tricuspic valve
    D. Pulmonary valve.

    229.

230. The function of a heart valve is to:
    A. Control blood flow
    B. Ensure that blood flows in one direction only
    C. Prevent overfilling of a chamber
    D. Maintain blood pressure.

    230.

231. Which of the following valve abnormalities may occur in rheumatic carditis?
    A. Simple narrowing
    B. Yellowish vegetations
    C. Fibrosis
    D. All of the above.

    231.

232. Mitral stenosis is the most common form of rheumatic valvular heart disease and takes years to develop. The result of mitral stenosis is that:
    A. Less blood flows into the left ventricle
    B. To maintain blood flow into the left ventricle, the left atrial pressure is increased
    C. Eventually pulmonary oedema occurs
    D. All of the above.

    232.

233. James now shows signs of congestive cardiac failure. Which of the following   233.
     positions is he likely to find most comfortable?
     A. Lying with one pillow
     B. Supported by pillows in the sitting position
     C. Supported by pillows in the sitting position with arms resting on a
        bedtable
     D. Supported by pillows in the sitting position with a knee pillow to
        prevent slipping.

234. Which of the following vital functions must be measured and recorded   234.
     regularly?
     A. Temperature, pulse rate and rhythm and blood pressure
     B. Pulse and respiration rates and temperature
     C. Temperature, respirations and blood pressure
     D. Pulse rate and rhythm, respiration rate and blood pressure.

235. James will be given digitalis. The effect of digitalis is to: 235.
     A. Increase the heart rate and weaken contractions
     B. Slow the heart rate and strengthen contractions
     C. Decrease cardiac output
     D. Decrease renal blood flow.

James is now in congestive cardiac failure.

True/false questions

The following questions (236–241) all refer to the nursing management of congestive cardiac failure. They are all of the true/false type. Consider each statement and decide whether you think it is true or false.

236. Digitalis toxicity causes arrhythmia.   236.

237. The apex heart beat must be obtained before administering digitalis.   237.

238. Digitalis causes anuria.   238.

239. Fluid intake and urinary output must be recorded carefully.   239.

240. Reduction of salt intake is unnecessary.   240.

241. Daily weighing indicates effectiveness of treatment and adjustment to   241.
     diuretic dosages.

Accurate monitoring of the patient's blood pressure is important in the nursing care of congestive cardiac failure. The following questions (242–247) relate to this procedure. They are all of the true/false type.

242. The patient should be at rest.   242.

243. The room should not be too warm or too cold.   243.

244. The sphygmomanometer cuff size is not important.   244.

245. The first sounds heard as cuff pressure is lowered indicates the systolic 245.
     pressure.

246. The complete disappearance of sounds indicates the diastolic pressure. 246.

247. It is more difficult to obtain accurate readings in obese patients.   247.

One or the most important therapeutic measures in severe heart failure is the administration of oxygen. Questions 248–256 relate to this therapy. They are all of the true/false type.

248. In severe heart failure oxygen saturation of the blood is reduced due to pulmonary congestion and stagnant hypoxia. | 248.

249. In pulmonary oedema high concentrations of oxygen should be given. | 249.

250. Oxygen administered via a nasal catheter at a flowrate of 5 to 7 litres per minute provides a mean concentration of 30 to 50 per cent. | 250.

251. A face mask is not efficient in providing an adequate concentration of oxygen. | 251.

252. An oxygen tent is not an efficient method of administering oxygen. | 252.

253. Oxygen administered via a nasal catheter can only be tolerated for a few hours. | 253.

254. Fire and explosions are more likely to occur when free oxygen is available. | 254.

255. To prevent an explosion and fire, only the patient must be prevented from smoking. | 255.

256. Environmental oxygen concentration is measured with a flowmeter. | 256.

Cardiac arrest can occur in a person previously apparently healthy as well as in one whose heart is diseased. The nurse should be able to recognize signs of cardiac arrest and be able to take action.

The following questions (257–264) relate to cardiac arrest. They are all of the true/false type.

257. In cardiac arrest pulses are absent. | 257.

258. There is absence of breathing. | 258.

259. Pupils are constricted. | 259.

260. The nurse should place the patient in the supine position. | 260.

261. External cardiac compressions are done using rhythmic pressure on the sternum 10 to 15 times per minute.

261.

262. Ventilation should be started immediately.

262.

263. Tissue anoxia for more than 4 to 6 minutes results in irreversible brain damage.

263.

264. In mouth-to-mouth resuscitation the cycle is repeated approximately 20 times per minute for adults and 12 times per minute for children.

264.

Acute juvenile rheumatism (rheumatic fever) answers and explanations (Questions 185 to 264)

Multiple choice *(Page 19)*

185. **A** The nurse should quickly make an assessment of the child's general condition and then decide on the best method to use for his admission.

186. **A** The amount of pain and his ability to move will determine the extent of handling he can tolerate. Some children may feel pain when being lifted or moved and it is important that he should be handled gently and with the minimum of disturbance to him. At this stage he will not be encouraged to walk (C).

187. **B** If he has painful joints, then a bedcage will be necessary to prevent the weight of the bedclothes further increasing discomfort.

188. **A** His temperature should be taken first before a bath is given. The pulse and breathing rate can be observed at the same time and should also be done before a bath or any activity is carried out. At this age the temperature is usually taken in the axilla. However, if a rectal temperature is requested the pulse and breathing rates are taken separately.

189. **B** A bedbath would be advisable. It prevents excessive movement and if done gently should not cause pain.

190. **C** Since drug dosage is based on the child's weight, it is important to ensure an accurate weight is obtained.

191. **C** Parents should be interviewed by nursing staff so that a profile of personality, likes and dislikes are obtained. This is useful in preparing a nursing care plan based on the child's needs.

192. **D** It is essential that either the doctor or the nurse establishes through questioning whether the child has been in contact with any infectious disease. This is to protect other ill children who are very susceptible to infection and for whom complications can have serious consequences. It is also helpful to know what relationships James has with other children, so that he can be placed near others of similar temperament. Likes and dislikes should be ascertained since it is important to recognize the child as an individual.

193. **D** The tonsils and the nose are the best regions for obtaining a swab. Each contains lymphoid tissue which acts as the first line of defence.

194. **C** A ten-year-old boy can be reasoned with and generally, once the procedure has been explained to him, will co-operate. However, it is still necessary to hold his head and hands since reflexly he may move his head and try to prevent the application of the swab, but it is not necessary to have him lying flat.

195. **B** It is not enough simply to touch the tonsillar region, but since the swabbing causes gagging, it should be carried out gently and quickly.

196. **C** Bacteriological investigation is required because it is necessary to
and   establish (i) presence and (ii) type of organisms and (iii) to establish
197. **D** sensitivity to various antibiotics and chemotherapeutic substances.

198. **C** Haemolytic streptococci is the commonest cause of throat infection. It produces many toxins which cause specific diseases. For example, the erythrogenic toxin causes rash in scarlet fever. Acute juvenile rheumatism is due to an allergic response to the toxin. The effect is delayed and therefore it is not generally apparent until some time after the initial streptococcal infection. Streptococcus viridans does not produce a soluble toxin. It is found in septic lesions of the teeth and gums and tends to invade already damaged tissue. When the heart valves are already damaged by the toxin of the Beta-haemolytic streptococcus, this may lead to sub-acute bacterial endocarditis.

199. **C** Blood analysis would establish that the child is anaemic. Anaemia can occur due to the action of toxins on the red blood cells causing haemolysis. It would also indicate raised white blood cell level.

200. **D** An X-ray of chest might demonstrate cardiac enlargement as evidence of cardiac involvement and an electrocardiogram would indicate abnormal heart activity. Measurement of the erythrocyte sedimentation rate is routinely carried out.

201. **A** The erythrocyte sedimentation rate is raised in infection, as well as in inflammatory disease and in malignancy. Measurement of the ESR is a non-specific screening test and is useful in assessing progress or deterioration.

202. **C** Salicylates are antipyretic and anti-inflammatory as well as analgesic (relieving pain) in action. Salicylates in the form of aspirin is the drug generally chosen and should give relief within 24 hours.

203. **C** Penicillin is effective against haemolytic streptococcus and is the drug generally given. Sulphadiazine is also effective but is not usually prescribed when administration over a prolonged period is required.

204. **D** Tinnitus, deafness, vomiting, nausea and hyperventilation are signs of toxicity. In children, hyperventilation can result in respiratory alkalosis which is followed by metabolic acidosis. Aspirin also causes gastro-intestinal irritation and may lead to bleeding.

205. **B** Penicillins are potent sensitizers and allergic reactions are not uncommon. It is therefore important to ask the parents if James has had previous treatment with the drug, and if there was any abnormal allergic reaction. Because of the danger of anaphylactic shock, patients who are hypersensitive should not be given penicillin. When the results of the swab are received, another antibiotic will have to be prescribed if the infecting organism proves to be insensitive to penicillin.

206. **D** All of the options may well be present but skin rashes are the most common features and can include urticaria, macula, papula or purpuric rashes.

207. **D** Corticosteroids are useful because of their anti-inflammatory, anti-allergic and lympholytic properties. However, they have several side-effects which include all the options mentioned. There is redistribution of fat, growth in children is impeded because of the inhibitory effect on protein synthesis, and there is an increased susceptibility of infection because of the action on lymphocytes.

208. **A** Initially bedrest is considered essential, particularly during the acute arthritic stage or if carditis is evident. It is also considered necessary if chorea develops. This may occur as an inflammatory complication of haemolytic streptococcal infection involving the central nervous system.

209. **D** 4-hourly measurements are usually adequate in dealing with any change in the child's condition. The sleeping pulse rate is an important observation which will provide information of cardiac function.

210. **D** A ripple bed is useful, though some children find it uncomfortable initially. Where possible limited movement and frequent turning can be encouraged to ease pressure on the dependent parts.

211. **A** If the child is unable or reluctant to eat, fluids only should be given. Once he feels inclined to eat he can be introduced gradually to a normal diet. It is important to keep the child well hydrated to enable the body, and particularly the kidney tissue, to function properly.

212. **C** A fluid chart records both intake and output. The output is primarily urine, though other fluid loss such as vomitus is also measured and recorded. A balance between fluid intake and output indicates the efficiency of the kidneys. Accuracy in measurement is essential.

213. **D** Soluble aspirin is often better tolerated than ordinary aspirin. Giving milk with it may also help to avoid gastric irritation.

214. **C** It is a noise heard over areas of the cardiovascular system where blood flow is turbulent. This type of flow can occur whether valves are normal or abnormal. Both systolic and diastolic murmurs can be heard. In mitral incompetence the murmur occurs throughout the entire systolic phase.

215. **C** A persistently raised sleeping pulse rate is an early indication of cardiac involvement and may be due to toxins. Arrhythmia may or may not be present at the same time. It is due to inflammatory processes of the A–V node.

216. **B** Although all three coats of the heart may be affected, the endocardium, myocardium and the mitral valve are most likely to be affected.

217. **C** Prednisone is less inclined to cause salt and water retention than other steroids, but sodium intake is often restricted. There is increased glucose formation from protein giving increased availability of carbohydrate. This leads to redistribution of fat with increased deposition in the face and other areas. It is important therefore to control the carbohydrate intake.

218. **C** This range is considered normal for a boy of ten, with a mean of 91.

219. **A** It is advisable to increase his activity gradually and to prevent excessive exertion which would require greater cardiac effort. It is also true though that children of that age recognize their limits, but it is the nurse's responsibility to assess the child's response to activity and set limits in order to protect him.

220. **C** Measurement of pulse rate and rhythm should be done before, during and after mobility. This will provide information about the heart's ability to cope with increased demands.

True/false *(Page 26)*

221. **True** Many authorities believe that to prevent further streptococcal infection and to reduce the risk of a relapse, it is worthwhile to give penicillin prophylactically until 18 years of age. In some cases it may be necessary to give the penicillin as a monthly intramuscular dose to ensure that the drug is taken.

222. **True** A programme of possible activity should be discussed with the parents but it should be stressed that the child should not be regarded as an invalid.

223. **False** Some restrictions should be placed on his activity, e.g. games like football would be too strenuous.

224. **False** It is advisable that the child should adjust to his home environment before returning to school.

225. **False** If his prednisone has been discontinued, then he can be given a normal diet.

226. **False** Isolation is not necessary, but care should be taken not to expose him unnecessarily to infection.

227. **True** The child should continue to attend the hospital outpatient department at regular intervals. The general practitioner will be sent all the information regarding hospital findings and treatment. Guidance will be given regarding future management.

228. **True** It is advisable that both penicillin and streptomycin should be given when major dental work is required. This is to prevent infection by the streptococcus viridans which attacks already damaged tissue and leads to vegetative growths on the mitral valve.

Multiple choice *(Page 27)*

229. **B** The mitral valve is most commonly involved, the aortic valve often, while the tricuspid and pulmonary valves are less frequently affected. Initially there may be oedema of the valve and thickening with yellowish vegetation leading to fusion and retraction of cusps. Eventually the valves become stenosed and functional changes, such as regurgitation, occur.

230. **B** The valves are so constructed that when the ventricles contract the increasing pressure of the ventricular blood closes the valves. The valves are prevented from being forced into the atria by the action of the chordae tendinae.

231. **D** See answer 229.

232. **D** Stenosis of the mitral valve prevents sufficient blood from entering the left ventricle and to maintain blood flow, left atrial pressure is increased. This increased pressure is reflected into the pulmonary veins and capillaries. As stenosis progresses, pulmonary oedema appears. Dyspnoea is often acute during exertion.

233. **C** This is probably the most comfortable position and allows for maximum lung expansion. A knee pillow may interfere with venous return.

234. **D** Increase and decrease in rate with arrhythmia should be recognized and reported. Blood pressure increase can lead to cardiovascular accident.

235 **B** Digitalis suppresses ventricular arrhythmias, increases venous tone, increases renal blood flow and slows the heart rate. Its primary action is to strengthen myocardial contractions causing the heart to beat more slowly and to greater effect.

True/false *(Page 29)*

236. **True** This is due to the drug's direct effect on the A–V node causing a prolonged P–R time which can lead to complete heart block.

237. **True** This is essential to detect excessive slowing of the heart rate and arrhythmia and determines advisability of giving subsequent doses.

238. **False** Since digitalis increases renal blood flow, it has a mild diuretic effect and there will be increased urinary output.

239. **True** This must be carried out accurately as an indication of renal function and as evidence of fluid loss where oedema is a cardinal feature.

240. **False** Salt intake should be restricted, i.e. no salt should be added to the food. This is particularly important where water is retained and oedema is evident.

241. **True** As stated. This is related to the presence of oedema.

242. **True** When recording blood pressure it is the resting pressure which is generally required.

243. **True** Extremes of room temperature can affect blood pressure measurements.

244. **False** It is important to use the correct size of cuff. Different sizes are available, e.g. for infants, small children and various adult sizes. The cuff should not extend beyond the elbow as this would obliterate the pulse.

245. **True** As stated.

246. **False** A sudden fall in the intensity of the sounds indicates diastolic pressure—faint sounds may persist indefinitely.

247. **True** Greater cuff pressure is needed to occlude the artery. In this case, to get a valid measurement a wider cuff should be used.

248. **True**   Pulmonary congestion prevents perfusion of gases and leads to decreased oxygen saturation of the blood, while inadequate blood flow through the tissues leads to stagnant hypoxia. Congestion is due to increased pulmonary venous pressure with fluid escaping from the pulmonary capillaries into the interstitial spaces and alveoli with consequent alveolar collapse.

249. **True**   High concentrations of inspired oxygen increase the diffusion gradient between the alveoli and the blood. It also helps to prevent serum from passing through the vessel wall by exerting pressure on the pulmonary epithelium during expiration. It is important to remember that inspired oxygen concentrations exceeding 80% have significant toxic effects on the alveolar capillary endothelium and bronchi and should not be given over long periods. Concentrations of inspired oxygen of less than 60% are usually well tolerated for long periods without obvious toxicity.

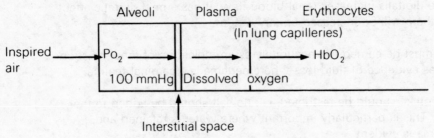

PULMONARY OEDEMA

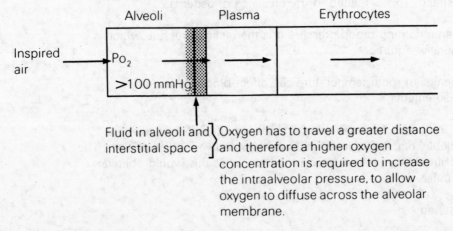

Fluid in alveoli and interstitial space } Oxygen has to travel a greater distance and therefore a higher oxygen concentration is required to increase the intraalveolar pressure, to allow oxygen to diffuse across the alveolar membrane.

250. **True**   As stated.

251. **False**   A tight-fitting mask is capable of delivering up to 100% inspired oxygen. There are a variety of face masks available and the flow of oxygen required for a given percentage is predetermined by the mask design.

252. **False** Provided the plastic is well tucked in preventing loss of oxygen then it is an efficient method of oxygen administration. When the tent is frequently opened the inflow of oxygen should be increased.

253. **False** Oxygen given via a nasal catheter can be maintained over quite a long time, but it may be necessary to decrease the inflow. Nasal catheters are not normally used for children, who do not seem to tolerate them well.

254. **True** As stated.

255. **False** Everyone attending the patient or working in the vicinity where oxygen is used must be fully aware of the danger of fire.

256. **False** Environmental (inspired) oxygen concentration is monitored with an oximeter. Frequent readings must be taken to prevent a build-up of oxygen concentration in the environment above the recommended level. In young children the inspired oxygen concentration may be between 25% to 35%, although higher concentrations may be given under controlled conditions. High inspired oxygen concentrations given over a prolonged period can cause damage to alveolar capillary endothelium and bronchi, while in pre-term infants it can damage retinal vessels.

257. **True** Absent or inadequate heart contractions are manifested clinically by absent pulse.

258. **True** Respiratory arrest may be secondary to cardiac arrest.

259. **False** Pupils are dilated due to lack of perfusion of the brain. This will occur when the circulation ceases as a result of absent or inadequate cardiac contractions.

260. **True** To initiate cardiac and respiratory resuscitation the patient must be placed in a suitable position which is accepted as the supine position. Assistance should be sought as soon as possible.

261. **False** Chest compressions should be done at a rate of 60 to 70 per minute. If two operators are present, one should interpose a breath between every five chest compressions provided by the other.

262. **False** Before starting ventilation it is essential to ensure that the airway is clear.

263. **True** If blood flow to the brain stops, consciousness is lost in 5 to 10 seconds causing irreparable brain damage within 5 to 10 minutes. Brain tissue has a high metabolic rate and without oxygen store it cannot tolerate hypoxia.

264. **False** The cycle is repeated approximately 12 times per minute for adults and 20 times per minute for children.

Anaemia

The following questions (265–308) are based on the case history given below:

Mrs Jennifer Graham is 34 years old, happily married with three children aged 6 years, 4 years and 18 months. She is always tired. This tiredness started about a year ago and in the last few weeks she has experienced dizzy spells. She thought her tiredness was a result of coping with her home and young family and it was not until she actually fainted that she considered going to see her doctor.

The doctor, noticing her apprehension and pale complexion, checked up on her obstetric history. Apart from some early morning sickness, her first two pregnancies had been normal but when her last little girl was born she had a fairly severe post-partum haemorrhage and she remembers being given a blood transfusion. For the last year she has had heavy menstrual periods. The doctor's provisional diagnosis was anaemia and he asked Mrs Graham if she would make arrangements to have the children cared for so that she could be admitted to hospital for investigation.

On admission, Mrs Graham was pale, her temperature was 36°C, pulse rate 98 and respiration rate 26 per minute.

Multiple choice questions

The following questions (265–269) are all of the multiple choice type. Read the questions and from the possible answers select ONE which you think is correct.

265. The term anaemia means:
    A. A deficiency in the quality of the red blood cells
    B. A deficiency in the quantity of the red blood cells
    C. Neither of the above
    D. Both of the above.

265.

266. There are several possible causes of anaemia. In Mrs Graham's case the cause was likely to be:
    A. Increased destruction of red blood cells
    B. Diminished production of red blood cells
    C. Blood loss
    D. All of the above.

266.

267. The type of anaemia resulting from chronic blood loss is called: 267.
    A. Iron deficiency
    B. Pernicious
    C. Haemolytic
    D. Aplastic.

268. In iron deficiency anaemia the red blood cells are: 268.
    A. Decreased in number
    B. Small in size (microcytic)
    C. Pale in colour (hypochromic)
    D. All of the above.

269. This type of anaemia is most common: 269.
    A. In the aged
    B. In young women
    C. In young men
    D. In the middle-aged of both sexes.

Mrs Graham's history was recorded and she was examined by the doctor.

True/false questions

Questions 270–289 relate to the clinical features which the doctor might expect to find when examining a patient with a provisional diagnosis of iron deficiency anaemia. They are all of the true/false type and consist of a number of statements, some of which are true and some of which are false. Consider each statement and decide whether you think it is true or false.

The following signs and symptoms may be present:

270. Clubbed fingers with soft nails	270.
271. A pale, sweaty skin	271.
272. Roughened tongue	272.
273. Inflammation of the corners of the mouth	273.
274. Increased appetite and body weight	274.
275. Indigestion	275.
276. Breathless on exertion with palpitations.	276.

Several of these signs and symptoms were found by the doctor when he examined Mrs Graham. He therefore arranged for the following investigations to be carried out to confirm his diagnosis of iron-deficiency anaemia.

277. Haemoglobin estimation   277.

278. Red blood cell count   278.

279. Marrow puncture   279.

280. Schilling test   280.

281. Gastric acid secretion test   281.

282. Barium meal   282.

283. Respiratory function test.   283.

True/false questions

Questions 284–289 refer to results of blood examination. Indicate whether the statements are true or false.

284. Haemoglobin levels in men are generally lower than in women   284.

285. The normal haemoglobin level in young women is from 10.6 to   285.
      12.0 g per 100 ml

286. Haemoglobin levels rarely fall below 8 g per 100 ml   286.

287. The normal red blood cell count for an adult is approximately   287.
      5 000 000 per mm^3

288. The normal white blood cell count for an adult is 200 000 per mm^3 288.

289. The normal platelet count for an adult is 5–10 000 per mm^3.   289.

The results of Mrs Graham's test showed that her haemoglobin level was only 4 g per 100 ml and her red bloodcell count was also well below normal. This confirmed the doctor's diagnosis.

When taking Mrs Graham's personal history, the doctor had learnt that Mr Graham had been made redundant over a year ago and was still unemployed. To help the family budget Mrs Graham had taken a part-time job. But as she became increasingly tired and unwell she had to give it up. This meant that they were no longer able to buy the type of food which they had been used to. Her anaemia was therefore due not only to her chronic blood loss but also to a deficiency of iron in her diet.

Multiple choice questions
The following questions (290–298) are all of the multiple choice type. Read the questions and from the possible answers select the ONE which you think is correct.

290. For women of menstrual age the normal daily iron requirements are:
    A. 6 mg
    B. 12 mg
    C. 18 mg
    D. 24 mg.

290.

291. Which one of the following groups of people is *least* likely to have a deficiency of iron in the blood?
    A. Patients suffering from achlorhydria
    B. Pregnant women
    C. Lactating women
    D. One-month-old infants.

291.

292. All of the following contain iron. Which is the richest and most easily absorbed source?
    A. Red meat
    B. Eggs
    C. Beans
    D. Bread.

292.

293. Which one of the following substances is necessary for the formation of haemoglobin?
    A. Calcium
    B. Calciferol
    C. Carotene
    D. Cyanocobalamin.

293.

Because Mrs Graham's haemoglobin level was very low it was
decided to give her a period of complete bed rest.

---

294. The main reason for prescribing bed rest was: 294.
    A. Low level of sugar in the blood
    B. Low level of oxygen in the blood
    C. Loss of weight
    D. Overwork.

295. Mrs Graham's mouth will require attention. Care should be given: 295.
    A. Night and morning
    B. Before and after meals
    C. As requested by the patient
    D. At regular intervals.

296. Her nails must be kept short to prevent them from becoming: 296.
    A. Clubbed
    B. Spoonshaped
    C. Ingrowing
    D. Infected.

297. Mrs Graham's skin must be cared for. In her case the treatment would be to   297.
use:
    A. Methylated spirit
    B. Soap and water
    C. An emollient lotion
    D. Talcum powder.

298. When considering Mrs Graham's menu, she should be encouraged to eat: 298.
    A. What she feels like
    B. Spicy meals to stimulate the flow of saliva
    C. Only bland milky foods
    D. Plenty of green vegetables.

True/false questions

The following questions (299–306) are of the true/false type. Indicate whether the statements are true or false.

As soon as the diagnosis was confirmed, Mrs Graham was prescribed a course of iron.

---

299. Parenteral iron therapy is given in preference to oral.   299.

300. Iron given by mouth may irritate the gastrointestinal mucosa.   300.

301. Oral iron should always be given before meals.   301.

302. Ferrous sulphate 200 mgs three times a day is the commonest way of prescribing iron.   302.

303. Constipation is a common complication during iron therapy.   303.

304. The black coloration of the stools of patients receiving iron therapy denotes the presence of altered blood.   304.

305. Parenteral iron therapy must be given by deep intramuscular injection.   305.

306. A blood transfusion is always given before starting iron therapy.   306.

Mrs Graham responded well to bed rest and she tolerated the oral iron. There was no need to give her a blood transfusion.

Multiple choice questions
Questions 307 and 308 are of the multiple choice type. Read the questions and from the possible answers select the ONE which you think is correct.

307. At the start of treatment her haemoglobin levels were checked: 307.
    A. Four-hourly
    B. Twice daily
    C. Daily
    D. Weekly.

308. The level was found to rise by: 308.
    A. One per cent per day
    B. One per cent per week
    C. Five per cent per day
    D. One hundred per cent per week.

Once an increase in her haemoglobin level had been established, Mrs Graham was told she could leave hospital and continue her therapy at home. Before she left she was seen by the dietitian, who explained which foods were the best sources of iron and how she could plan the family meals on a reduced budget and still maintain her daily iron requirement.

She was given a supply of iron tablets and an out-patient appointment was made for four weeks' time, when her haemoglobin level would again be checked.

Anaemia answers and explanations

Multiple choice *(Page 40)*

265. **D** The term anaemia may be defined as a state in which the quantity or quality of the circulating red cells is reduced below the normal level.

266. **C** Anaemia can result from A, B and C but in Mrs Graham's case it was due to blood loss from her heavy periods over the past twelve months.

267. **A** Chronic blood loss results in iron deficiency anaemia (A).

    Pernicious anaemia (B) is due to the absence of the intrinsic factor in the stomach. This factor is necessary for the absorption of vitamin B_{12} from the gastrointestinal tract. Vitamin B_{12} is essential for the formation of red blood corpuscles in the bone marrow.

    Haemolytic anaemia (C) is due to the excessive breakdown of red blood cells. There are several causes of this condition, one of which is an incompatible blood transfusion.

    Aplastic anaemia (D) is when no red blood cells are being produced in the red bone marrow.

268. **D** Red blood cells are reduced in number. They are microcytic in type having diameters below the normal range. They are hypochromic due to a diminished content of haemoglobin.

269. **B** Iron deficiency anaemia is more common in women than in men. Its occurrence is greater during a woman's fertile years due to menstruation and childbirth.

    Iron deficiency anaemia may occur in men and women at any age when it is frequently due to poor diet or to blood loss from other sources, e.g. bleeding haemorrhoids.

True/false *(Page 44)*

270. **False** Nails tend to become dry and brittle. In 28% of patients with iron deficiency anaemia, nails become thin and spoon-shaped. This condition is known as koilonychia.

271. **False** These patients have a dry skin. While pallor is often present, many people are naturally pale, therefore this is not always the most reliable picture. Pale conjunctiva of the eyes is a more reliable sign.

272. **False** The tongue becomes sore and red with loss of papillae giving it a smooth, shiny appearance.

273. **True** Many patients complain of sores or cracks at the corners of the mouth (angular stomatitis).

274. **False** The appetite is invariably poor. If the anaemia continues untreated, there is a subsequent loss of weight.

275. **False** Indigestion is not usually a symptom of iron deficiency anaemia.

276. **True** Breathlessness and palpitations are both common symptoms of anaemia. Respirations increase in an effort to get more oxygen into the lungs and the heart beats faster in an effort to get more oxygen to the tissues. These symptoms are more marked when muscular activity is increased.

277. **True** Haemoglobin estimation is carried out. The haemoglobin level is reduced in iron deficiency anaemia.

278. **True** Due to Mrs Graham's history of heavy menstrual bleeding, her red blood cell count would be carried out.

279. **False** Peripheral blood is examined in the diagnosis of iron deficiency anaemia. A marrow puncture biopsy is carried out as a diagnostic investigation in pernicious (vitamin B_{12} deficiency) anaemia, white blood cell abnormality and disease of the bone marrow.

280. **False** A Schilling test is carried out to investigate vitamin B_{12} deficiency anaemia.

281. **True** A gastric acid secretion test is carried out to determine the presence or absence of hydrochloric acid in the stomach. Hydrochloric acid is necessary for the absorption of iron from foodstuff.

282. **False** A barium meal is carried out to investigate the presence of a gastric abnormality, e.g. peptic ulcer or gastric carcinoma. Bleeding from either condition can cause iron deficiency anaemia. It is unlikely that Mrs Graham would be given a barium meal as it is known that she has very heavy periods.

283. **False** Respiratory function tests are used to detect respiratory abnormality. Mrs Graham's breathlessness is due to a low haemoglobin level with a low oxygen carrying power and not to respiratory disease.

284. **False** Haemoglobin levels are slightly higher in men. The mean average is 15.6 g per 100 ml of blood.

285. **False** The normal haemoglobin levels for young women range from 11.5–16.4 g per 100 ml of blood.

      The mean average is 13.7 g per 100 ml of blood.

286. **True**   Medical help is usually sought before haemoglobin levels fall as low as 8 g per 100 ml of blood. Signs and symptoms of iron deficiency anaemia with this level of haemoglobin would be very marked.

287. **True**   The normal red blood cell count for an adult is 5 000 000 per mm^3 of blood.

288. **False**   The normal white blood cell count for an adult is 5000 to 10 000 per mm^3 of blood.

289. **False**   The normal platelet count for an adult is 200 000 per mm^3 of blood approximately.

Multiple choice *(Page 45)*

290. **C**   The normal daily iron requirements for a woman of menstrual age is 18 mg.

291. **D**   Iron is stored in the liver of the developing fetus. This iron is utilized after birth, during the period of milk feeding, as milk is deficient in iron.

292. **A**   Red meat is the richest and most easily absorbed source of iron.

293. **D**   Cyanocobalamin (vitamin B$_{12}$), a substance present in liver, meat, milk, eggs and cheese, is necessary in the diet for the formation of haemoglobin. Calcium (A) is essential for the clotting of blood.

294. **B**   Muscular activity makes demands on the reduced oxygen level to body tissue and in particular to the vital centres in iron deficiency anaemia. Bed rest reduces this extra demand and will conserve the patient's strength.

295. **D**   Frequent, gentle oral hygiene given at regular intervals is necessary to prevent infection of the mouth. It will also make food more palatable.

296. **D**   Nails must be kept short by careful clipping. The dry, brittle nails may crack and tear with the possible risk of infection of the nailbed (D). Cutting will not prevent the spoon-shaped formation (B). Clubbed nails (A) are a sign of respiratory dysfunction.

297. **C**   While it is necessary to keep the skin clean with soap and water (B), the application of an emollient lotion is soothing to the dry skin and prevents it from cracking. Methylated spirit (A) would make the skin even drier.

298. **D** Green vegetables contribute valuable amounts of iron if they are eaten regularly. Initially it is much better to assist Mrs Graham in her choice of menu. This guides her in selecting foods which give good sources of iron.

True/false *(Page 47)*

299. **False** Parenteral iron therapy should be used only when iron given by the oral route cannot be tolerated. This may be due to gastric irritation or when a disorder of the gastro-intestinal tract prevents the proper absorption of iron.

300. **True** Patients receiving oral iron therapy may experience gastro-intestinal upsets such as nausea, vomiting, abdominal pain and disorders of bowel function.

301. **False** Oral iron therapy given after the ingestion of food reduces the risk of irritation to the gastric mucosa.

302. **True** The most common form of iron prescribed is ferrous sulphate in doses of 200 mg three times a day. It is the cheapest, easiest and safest method of administering iron.

303. **True** Diarrhoea or constipation may occur with the administration of oral iron, but constitpation is by far the commonest problem.

304. **False** Unwanted iron is excreted by the colon. It is the presence of this iron which gives the black coloration to the stools in the administration of iron. When the patient is having iron she must be warned about passing black coloured stools in order to prevent unnecessary worry.

    Altered blood in the stool can also cause black coloration. This stool has an unmistakable characteristic odour.

305. **True** Parenteral iron therapy must be given deep into the muscle to prevent staining of the skin which may last for several months and to prevent discomfort in the area of the injection. After withdrawing of the needle, the injection site must not be rubbed.

    The patient must be observed for adverse reactions and signs of iron toxicity such as nausea and faintness.

306. **False** Not all patients suffering from iron deficiency anaemia require a blood transfusion. Most improve with a diet rich in iron and with oral iron therapy. A blood transfusion is given when the iron deficiency is very severe and haemoglobin levels are extremely low (below 5 g per 100 ml of blood).

Multiple choice *(Page 48)*

307. **C** In the early stages haemoglobin levels will be checked daily to observe
the effect of the treatment being given. Later, when the blood picture
improves the haemoglobin will be checked weekly until Mrs Graham
leaves hospital. After that she will have monthly checks for a period of
six months.

308. **A** Effective iron therapy should lead to an increase of one per cent per day.

Hypertension

The following questions (309–378) are based on the case history given below. They are all of the multiple choice type. Read each question and from the possible answers select the ONE which you think is correct.

Mr Clifford Dowling, aged 56 years, and his wife, Hilda, live in a two-bedroomed maisonette on a Council estate. The maisonette is on the second floor in a block of similar dwellings and has a long flight of steps leading to the front door, with two further staircases inside (one leading to the living quarters and the second leading to the bedrooms).

Mrs Dowling is a trained nurse and follows part-time employment at the local hospital. Mr Dowling served for many years in the Royal Air Force, and since retiring from the Air Force has been employed as a business consultant. He is used to making decisions and giving instructions. He is also used to being obeyed!

The Dowlings are both very active people who take a keen interest in local affairs and their church. Most of their spare time is occupied with coffee mornings, bazaars and other fund-raising activities for the church. They have two children who are both married and living in different parts of the country.

For the past four years, Mr Dowling has had symptoms of essential hypertension. This has not worried him unduly and has not been of sufficient severity to warrant medical treatment.

309. Normal blood pressure for a healthy adult is within the range of:
    A.   90/50–120/70 mm Hg
    B. 110/60–150/85 mm Hg
    C. 130/80–170/100 mm Hg
    D. 150/85–180/120 mm Hg.

309.

310. The term 'blood pressure' describes the:
    A. Force by which blood is pushed through the arteries as the heart beats
    B. Permeability of the walls of the blood vessels
    C. Force by which blood from the veins is drawn into the atria of the heart
    D. Elasticity of the walls of the blood vessels.

310.

311. With reference to normal blood pressure, which of the following statements is true?
    A. In a healthy adult, it should remain at a constant level throughout life.
    B. In a healthy adult, the diastolic pressure should increase by about 10 mm Hg with each decade of life.
    C. It may be influenced by age, posture, exercise and emotion.
    D. It is usually low in people who have a fast pulse rate.

    311.

312. With reference to high blood pressure, which of the following statements is true?
    A. It is a common symptom of emotional shock
    B. It commonly causes the arteries to become dilated
    C. It may be caused by dilatation of the arteries
    D. It may be either a symptom of disease or a cause of disease.

    312.

313. The most common cause of high blood pressure is:
    A. Vasoconstriction
    B. Vasodilatation
    C. Valvular heart disease
    D. Varicose veins.

    313.

314. Which of the following would be most likely to cause a person's blood pressure to rise?
    A. Taking a cold shower
    B. Taking a hot bath
    C. Receiving a sudden fright
    D. Sunbathing.

    314.

315. Which of the following would be most likely to cause a person's blood pressure to fall?
    A. Lying down after being in the upright position
    B. Standing upright after being in the supine position
    C. Sitting down, reading a book
    D. Going for a long walk.

    315.

316. The most common symptoms of hypertension are:
    A. Pyrexia, tachycardia and giddiness
    B. Tachycardia, epistaxis and haematuria
    C. Headache, pyrexia and haematuria
    D. Headache, giddiness and epistaxis.

    316.

317. Which of the following statements most accurately describes the term
     'essential hypertension'?
     A. High blood pressure secondary to renal disease
     B. High blood pressure which does not respond to treatment with
        hypotensive drugs
     C. High blood pressure caused by the patient's excitable temperament
     D. High blood pressure for which no definite cause can be found.

317.

318. The term 'malignant hypertension' is used to describe a form of high blood
     pressure which:
     A. Occurs as a result of carcinoma with metastases
     B. Occurs in patients who have leukaemia
     C. Results in the patient developing sarcoma within a few years of the onset
        of symptoms
     D. Results in the patient's death within a few years of the onset of
        symptoms.

318.

319. The main difference between essential hypertension and malignant
     hypertension is that, malignant hypertension:
     A. Produces more severe symptoms in a shorter length of time
     B. Is secondary to disease of the vital organs
     C. Is a hereditary condition
     D. Responds to treatment with cytotoxic drugs.

319.

320. Hypertension commonly results in the patient developing heart failure. With
     reference to this, which part of the heart is likely to fail first?
     A. Right atrium
     B. Right ventricle
     C. Left atrium
     D. Left ventricle.

320.

Although Mr Dowling's hypertension has not been of sufficient
severity to warrant medical treatment, he has been visiting his
family practitioner every six months for a routine check of his
general condition. At his most recent visit, he told the doctor that
he had been experiencing pains in his chest at irregular intervals.
Mr Dowling described the pain as feeling like a tight band around
his chest. This pain he experienced on physical exertion. The doctor
diagnosed angina pectoris and gave Mr Dowling a prescription for
glyceryl trinitrate. He also advised Mr Dowling to avoid undue
stress and strenuous exercise.

321. Any of the following conditions may cause angina pectoris, but which one is   321.
     the *most common* cause?
     A. Aortic stenosis
     B. Aortic aneurysm
     C. Anaemia
     D. Arteriosclerosis.

322. Angina pectoris occurs as a direct result of: 322.
     A. A reduction in the blood supply to the muscle of the heart
     B. A reduction in the volume of blood passing through the chambers of the
        heart
     C. An increase in the volume of blood passing through the chambers of the
        heart
     D. A complete absence of the blood supply to a portion of the myocardium.

323. If the correct answer has been selected for question 322 this condition is   323.
     known as:
     A. Ischaemic heart disease
     B. Hypertrophy of the heart
     C. Coronary thrombosis
     D. Myocardial infarction.

324. Typically, the pain of angina pectoris occurs on exertion and improves after   324.
     resting. This is because:
     A. Increased effort causes constriction of the coronary arteries
     B. The heart beat is weak
     C. The sinoatrial node is not receiving sufficient stimulation
     D. The blood supply to the myocardium is inadequate for increased activity.

325. High blood pressure is another contributory factor in producing angina. This   325.
     is because hypertension causes:
     A. Enlargement of the heart
     B. Dilatation of the coronary vessels
     C. A reduction in the oxygen content of the blood
     D. A reduction in the prothrombin content of the blood.

326. The doctor prescribed tablets of glyceryl trinitrate 0.5 mg for Mr Dowling.   326.
     0.5 mg is equal to:
     A. 5 grams
     B. 50 grams
     C. 50 microgrammes
     D. 500 microgrammes.

327. When administering a tablet of glyceryl trinitrate the nurse should instruct the   327.
patient to:
   A. Crush the tablet in a tissue and inhale the vapour
   B. Allow the tablet to dissolve slowly under the tongue
   C. Swallow the tablet whole with a hot drink
   D. Drink at least 180 ml of water after taking the tablet.

328. In order for glyceryl trinitrate tablets to have the best effect, they should be   328.
taken:
   A. As soon as the patient wakens in the morning and directly before going to
      bed at night
   B. Three times a day after food
   C. An hour before the patient commences any physical activity
   D. Whenever chest pain occurs.

329. Glyceryl trinitrate relieves the symptoms of angina because it is: 329.
   A. An analgesic
   B. An antispasmodic
   C. A vasodilator
   D. A bronchodilator.

330. Which of the following statements most accurately describes the action of   330.
glyceryl trinitrate?
   A. By relieving pain, it causes the myocardium to relax and so increases the
      blood supply
   B. It increases the blood supply to the myocardium by relieving spasm of the
      coronary arteries
   C. It increases the blood supply to the myocardium by dilating the coronary
      arteries
   D. By dilating the bronchioles it allows more oxygen to enter the blood
      which stimulates the myocardium to work harder.

Mr Dowling considered his angina to be a warning that he must reduce some of his activities. He continued with his full-time employment and served on various committees but curtailed his fund-raising activities to some of the less strenuous tasks. One Saturday morning, approximately a year later, Mrs Dowling returned home from her morning's duty at the hospital and had difficulty opening the door of the sitting-room. Eventually she forced her way into the room and found her husband on the floor just behind the door. He was deeply unconscious. A small coffee table was overturned on the floor. The telephone had also fallen onto the floor.

Stifling her feeling of panic, Mrs Dowling took charge of the situation.

331. Which of the following should have been Mrs Dowling's first action?
    A. Turn her husband into the semiprone position
    B. Commence mouth-to-mouth resuscitation
    C. Commence external cardiac massage
    D. Take and record her husband's pulse.

331.

332. Having dealt with the priority in question 331, Mrs Dowling's next action should be to:
    A. Move the fallen furniture to a place of safety
    B. Bang on the floor to attract the attention of the neighbours in the ground floor maisonette
    C. Check that the telephone is in working order
    D. Open the windows to assist ventilation.

332.

333. Once help has arrived, which of the following is an essential action for Mrs Dowling to take before escorting her husband to hospital?
    A. Check that domestic appliances, such as cooker and iron, have been turned off
    B. Ensure that all windows are closed
    C. Take all of Mr Dowling's tablets with her for identification
    D. Lock the front door as she leaves the maisonette.

333.

Mr Dowling was taken by ambulance to the local hospital. During the journey Mrs Dowling felt dazed and confused, due to the speed with which events had happened. She was still uncertain about what had happened to her husband and could not be certain whether he had had a stroke or a heart attack.

On arrival at the hospital, Mr Dowling was taken to the resuscitation bay of the Accident and Emergency Department, where a diagnosis of myocardial infarction was confirmed.

Subsequently he was admitted to the Intensive Care Unit. Mr Dowling had regained consciousness while in the Accident and Emergency Department and was aware of what was happening when he was admitted to the unit.

334. When assessing the needs of a patient just admitted to hospital, which of the following considerations must take priority?

The patient's:
A. Personal preferences
B. State of mobility
C. Physical condition
D. Social background.

334.

335. Which of the following is the most important duty of the nurse in charge of the ward when talking to Mrs Dowling?
A. Ensure that she understands that she will not be able to have any preferential treatment, despite the fact that she is a trained nurse
B. Show respect for her position as a trained nurse by using technical terms when speaking to her
C. Talk to her about her husband's condition but omit explaining the ward routine as she will be fully aware of this
D. Speak to her in a sympathetic manner, carefully explaining details of treatment, ward routine, etc.

335.

336. Which of the following statements most accurately describes the term 'myocardial infarction'?
A. Death of part of the heart muscle due to lack of oxygenated blood
B. Inflammation of the lining of the heart due to increased pressure in the cardiac chambers
C. Failure of the right side of the heart to pump blood to the lungs
D. Failure of the left side of the heart to pump blood to the body.

336.

337. Myocardial infarction most commonly occurs as a direct result of a:
    A. Deep vein thrombosis
    B. Thrombosis of the coronary artery
    C. Thrombosis of the coronary vein
    D. Pulmonary embolism.

    337.

338. Mr Dowling was attached to a cardiac monitor. With reference to reading cardiac monitors which one of the following is it most important that the nurse be able to recognize?
    A. Sinus rhythm
    B. Atrial fibrillation
    C. Ventricular fibrillation
    D. Heart block.

    338.

339. While passing the bed of a patient attached to a cardiac monitor, a junior nurse notices an irregularity of the electrocardiograph tracing. The first action of the nurse should be to:
    A. Call to a more senior nurse for help
    B. Strike the patient's chest with a clenched fist
    C. Check the position of the electrodes (leads)
    D. Observe the general condition of the patient.

    339.

340. During Mr Dowling's first night in hospital he suffered a cardiac arrest. Which of the following statements most accurately describes the term 'cardiac arrest'?
    A. An absence of the heart beat for longer than one minute but less than three minutes
    B. A sudden cessation of the circulation in a patient who was not expected to die at that time
    C. The simultaneous failure of the circulatory system and the respiratory system of any person regardless of his/her age or previous clinical condition
    D. The apparent death of any seriously ill patient under the age of 65 years.

    340.

Mr Dowling was successfully resuscitated from his cardiac arrest but he was nursed on complete bed rest for the next two weeks. During this time he developed a deep vein thrombosis of the left leg and the doctor prescribed a course of treatment with anticoagulant drugs. Initially, Mr Dowling was given intravenous heparin and oral tablets of warfarin. The heparin was discontinued but Mr Dowling continued to receive tablets of warfarin for several weeks.

341. Which of the following complications is most likely to occur as a result of Mr Dowling's deep vein thrombosis?
    A. A cerebral embolus
    B. A pulmonary embolus
    C. A further myocardial infarction
    D. Renal failure.

341.

342. Which of the following statements provides the most probable explanation for the fact that Mr Dowling was not treated with anticoagulant drugs until he had developed the complication of a deep vein thrombosis?
    A. The initial infarct was not large enough to warrant treatment with these drugs
    B. Patients with a history of hypertension have a greater tendency to cerebro vascular accidents
    C. These drugs are generally more effective in the treatment of arterial thrombi
    D. These drugs are generally more effective in the treatment of venous thrombi.

342.

343. The purpose of giving anticoagulant drugs is to:
    A. Reduce the risk of further thrombi forming
    B. Dissolve the thrombus which has formed
    C. Dissolve the thrombus which has formed and prevent further thrombi from forming
    D. Prevent emboli from the original thrombus travelling in the blood stream.

343.

344. Anticoagulant drugs act by:
    A. Delaying the clotting time of the blood
    B. Speeding the clotting time of the blood
    C. Increasing the number of platelets in the blood
    D. Increasing the production of prothrombin.

344.

345. Which one of the following must the nurse be especially alert for when a patient is being treated with anticoagulant drugs?
    A. Hypertension
    B. Hypotension
    C. Haematuria
    D. Haemophilia.

345.

346. When caring for a patient who is receiving anticoagulant drugs, the nurse must be especially careful to observe the skin for:
    A. Pressure sores
    B. Signs of sepsis
    C. Pigmentation
    D. Bruises.

346.

347. Which of the following is the most important duty of the nurse when giving
     tablets of warfarin to a patient?
     To give the tablets:
     A. Before meals
     B. After meals
     C. At precisely the same time/times each day
     D. Only if the pulse is above 60 beats per minute.

347.

348. Which of the following statements provides the most probable explanation
     for the fact that Mr Dowling was initially treated with both heparin and
     warfarin, and the treatment was later changed to warfarin only?
     A. A combination of the two drugs provides a more rapid effect
     B. A greater concentration of the anticoagulant is required in the blood
        stream during the early stages of treatment
     C. Heparin enhances the action of warfarin
     D. Heparin has a more rapid effect than warfarin.

348.

Three weeks after his admission to hospital Mr Dowling was
transferred from the intensive care unit to a general medical ward.
His recovery had been further complicated by the fact that he had
developed congestive cardiac failure.

---

349. Which of the following are the most common symptoms of congestive
     cardiac failure?
     A. Acute chest pain, oedema of the dependent areas and bradycardia
     B. Acute chest pain, cyanosis and polyuria
     C. Dyspnoea, bradycardia and polyuria
     D. Oedema of the dependent areas, cyanosis and dyspnoea.

349.

350. Which of the following statements most accurately describes the term
     congestive cardiac failure?
     A. The right side of the heart fails to function properly, so causing
        congestion of the venous system
     B. The left side of the heart fails to function properly, so causing
        congestion of the lungs
     C. The lungs fail to function properly, so causing congestion of the right
        ventricle
     D. The left ventricle fails to function properly, so causing congestion of the
        arteries.

350.

351. In which of the following positions should a patient be nursed during the   351.
acute stage of congestive cardiac failure?
A. Recumbent
B. Left lateral
C. Upright
D. Three-quarters prone.

352. When a patient is being treated for congestive cardiac failure, it is most   352.
important that the diet should:
A. Have a high calorie (Joule) content
B. Be light and easily digestible
C. Contain a large amount of roughage
D. Contain a large amount of protein.

353. Patients with congestive cardiac failure are usually given a low salt diet.   353.
This is because:
A. The kidneys are unable to excrete salt properly
B. An excess of salt in the blood causes profuse sweating
C. Drugs normally given to the patient encourage the retention of salt
D. An excess of salt in the blood increases the risk of ischaemic heart
disease.

354. Which of the following foods would be most suitable to give to a patient   354.
whose salt intake is being restricted?
A. Boiled bacon
B. Grilled sausages
C. Poached haddock
D. Fried egg.

By the time Mr Dowling was transferred to the general ward, his
drug regime consisted of:

Digoxin 250 microgrammes twice daily,
Frusemide 40 mg daily,
Slow K 600 mg twice daily,
Warfarin as per separate anticoagulant chart.

355. Digoxin is effective in the treatment of congestive cardiac failure because it: 355.
A. Increases the size of the cardiac chambers
B. Increases the rate at which the cardiac chambers empty
C. Delays the conduction of cardiac impulses
D. Strengthens the walls of the ventricles.

356. 250 microgrammes is equal to:
    A. 25.0 milligrammes
    B. 2.50 milligrammes
    C. 0.25 milligrammes
    D. 0.025 milligrammes.

356.

357. Before administering a dose of digoxin the patient's pulse should be taken. Which of the following is the correct action for the nurse to take if the pulse is found to be 50 beats per minute?
    A. Give the drug and take the pulse again an hour later
    B. Give the drug and notify the nurse in charge of the ward that the pulse is slow
    C. Omit the drug and make a written note on the patient's treatment sheet
    D. Omit the drug and notify the nurse in charge of the ward.

357.

358. Which of the following observation charts should be maintained whenever a patient is being treated with frusemide?
    A. Four-hourly temperature, pulse and respiration
    B. Twice daily apex beat
    C. Twice daily blood pressure
    D. Fluid balance.

358.

359. Frusemide is a drug which is usually given early in the morning. The reason for this is because:
    A. Drugs which are given once daily are always given with the early morning drug round
    B. If given later in the day the patient's sleep may be disturbed by nocturnal diuresis
    C. This drug is most effective if taken when the metabolic rate is low
    D. Giving the drug early in the morning will allow time for the patient's condition to improve before night time.

359.

360. Patients who are being treated for congestive heart failure are frequently given tablets of Slow K because this drug:
    A. Enhances the action of digitalis
    B. Enhances the action of frusemide
    C. Replaces potassium which has been lost by increased diuresis
    D. Replaces sodium which has been lost by increased diuresis.

360.

After Mr Dowling was transferred to the general ward his routine nursing care included:

Daily bed bath,
Attention to pressure areas,
Gradually increasing activity,
Twice daily temperature, pulse, respiration and blood pressure,
Fluid balance chart,
Daily weight recording.

---

361. One day while bed bathing Mr Dowling, a junior nurse noticed four details which needed attention. Which one should take priority and be dealt with first?
    A. His toe nails were long and dirty
    B. The skin over the sacral area was red
    C. His feet and ankles were more oedematous than usual
    D. The patient became dyspnoeic when lying down.

361.

362. Which one of the following patients in the medical ward is *most* likely to develop pressure sores unless great care is taken?
    A. A patient who is receiving terminal nursing care for cancer and is having injections of morphine every 4 hours
    B. A patient who had a cerebrovascular accident three weeks ago and is now fully ambulant but incontinent of urine
    C. An elderly gentleman who has oedema of the feet and ankles and can only walk for short distances
    D. A fourteen-year-old boy with diabetes mellitus who has been admitted for assessment and stabilization.

362.

363. With reference to fluid balance charts, which of the following statements is true?
    A. Blood loss need never be recorded on the chart as this is not a normal form of excretion
    B. When giving oral fluids to a patient the nurse must remember that 180 ml water provides the body with a greater volume of fluid than 180 ml of tea, coffee or milk
    C. All fluid intake and output should be recorded on the chart, regardless of the source or amount
    D. Only fluids given as liquid medicines may be omitted from the chart as these are recorded in the Kardex.

363.

364. Which of the following is the correct action for the nurse to take when recording oral fluid intake for a patient?
    A. Ask the patient what he has drunk in the previous four hours and chart accordingly
    B. Record the amount of fluid in the intake column directly it has been poured
    C. Record the amount of fluid directly the patient has drunk it
    D. Leave a measured amount of fluid on the patient's locker and come back later to record it when the glass is empty.

364.

365. When measuring the contents of a bed pan, a nurse finds the amount of urine is not sufficient to reach the first graduation mark of the measuring jug. Which of the following is the correct action for the nurse to take?
    A. Add water to the urine and record half the measured amount of volume
    B. Estimate the amount of urine and write on the chart 'approximately' beside the estimated amount
    C. Indicate on the chart that urine has been passed by writing '+' or 'P.U.'
    D. Disregard the urine as the amount is too small to be significant.

365.

366. The most probable reason for weighing Mr Dowling each day was to:
    A. Ensure that he was receiving sufficient nourishment
    B. Ensure that he did not become obese
    C. Assess his response to anticoagulant drugs
    D. Assess his response to diuretic drugs.

366.

Sometimes patients with congestive cardiac failure develop ascites and/or hydrothorax.

---

367. Ascites is a term used to describe:
    A. A collection of fluid in the peritoneal cavity
    B. A collection of air in the abdominal cavity
    C. Free fluid in the pelvic cavity
    D. Inflammation of the peritoneum.

367.

368. Which of the following statements most accurately describes the term hydrothorax?
    A. Collapse of a lobe of the lung
    B. Consolidation of the base of the lung
    C. A collection of fluid in the pleural cavity
    D. Inability of the pleura to produce its natural serous fluid.

368.

369. The reason that ascites and hydrothorax are common complications of
     congestive cardiac failure is because:
     A. Increased venous pressure forces fluid into the tissues and this fluid may
        collect in different cavities of the body
     B. Increased cardiac output causes an excess of fluid in the arteries which
        places greater strain on the major organs
     C. The major organs of the body are deprived of an adequate supply of
        oxygen
     D. The major membranes of the body are deprived of an adequate supply of
        nourishment.

369.

370. When preparing a patient for a paracentesis abdominis, which of the
     following is the most important duty of the nurse?

     Ensure that the:
     A. Rectum is empty
     B. Urinary bladder is empty
     C. Umbilicus is clean
     D. Pubic and abdominal skin have been shaved.

370.

371. Patients with hydrothorax sometimes have a chest drain inserted which is
     attached to underwater seal drainage. When nursing a patient in this
     situation all of the following are important but which is *most important?*

     To ensure that the:
     A. Tube leading away from the patient is attached to the longer of the two
        tubes of the drainage bottle
     B. Fluid in the drainage bottle covers the distal end of the tube leading from
        the patient
     C. Patient's respirations are taken and recorded every half hour
     D. Patient is nursed in the upright position.

371.

372. With reference to the position of an underwater seal drainage bottle, the most
     important duty of the nurse is to ensure that the bottle is:
     A. Securely attached to the bed at all times
     B. Placed on a tray before standing it on the floor
     C. Never moved during nursing procedures
     D. Kept below the level of the lungs.

372.

373. If an underwater seal drainage bottle should accidently be knocked over and
     broken while in use, what should the nurse do first?
     A. Pour disinfectant over the spilt fluid
     B. Remove the broken glass to a place of safety
     C. Apply a clamp to the drainage tube
     D. Protect the end of the drainage tube with a sterile dressing.

373.

374. When a chest drain is removed from a patient the most important duty of the person removing the drain is to:
  A. Ensure that the wound is immediately sealed with an air-tight dressing
  B. Take and record the patient's pulse immediately before and after removing the drain
  C. Check the wound at frequent, regular intervals for signs of haemorrhage
  D. Encourage the patient to breathe deeply.

374.

Five weeks after his admission, Mr Dowling was discharged from hospital. He returned home and was cared for by his wife.

---

375. The following people should all be notified of Mr Dowling's discharge, but which one takes priority?
  A. His industrial medical officer
  B. His family practitioner
  C. The health visitor
  D. The outpatient appointments clerk.

375.

376. Mr Dowling was provided with hospital transport to take him home. The most important reason for this was because:
  A. His wife was unable to drive
  B. He had been very seriously ill
  C. He would find it very confusing to be among noisy traffic after a long period in hospital
  D. He would need a great deal of assistance to mount the many stairs leading to his maisonette.

376.

377. When a patient is provided with hospital transport for discharge from hospital, which of the following is the most important duty of the nurse?

  To ensure that:
  A. The relatives know the exact time of day the patient will be arriving
  B. The patient's personal possessions are all safely packed early in the morning
  C. Someone is in the house to receive the patient
  D. A friend or relative comes to the hospital to accompany the patient on the journey.

377.

378. The prognosis for patients with congestive cardiac failure is usually:
  A. Good, provided that the condition is not secondary to some other disease
  B. Good, provided that the patient receives medication for the rest of his life
  C. Poor, because treatment only relieves the symptoms but does not cure the condition
  D. Poor, because it is always secondary to left ventricular failure.

378.

Hypertension answers and explanations
(Questions 309–378)

309: **B** In a healthy adult the blood pressure is normally within the range of
110/60–150/85 mm Hg. Another way of expressing this is to say that
systolic pressure normally averages from 110 to 150 mm Hg, while
diastolic pressure normally averages from 60 to 85 mm Hg.

310. **A** Blood pressure is a term which is used to describe the force with which
blood is pushed through the arteries as the heart beats. When the heart
contracts, blood is pushed into the arteries and is at its maximum
pressure. This is known as systolic pressure. When the heart rests
between beats, blood in the arteries is at its lowest pressure and this is
known as diastolic pressure.

(A) is therefore a definition of blood pressure; (B), (C) and (D) are
factors affecting the pressure.

311. **C** When you turn on a tap, many factors are working together to influence
the pressure of water which flows: the amount of water in the tank, the
angle of the stopcock, the condition of the pipes. In the same way, many
factors in the body work together to influence the blood pressure: the
amount of blood circulating, the strength of the heart beat and the
condition of the blood vessels. From this it can be seen that blood
pressure may be influenced by age (the blood vessels lose their
elasticity); posture and exercise (greater effort is needed by the heart);
and emotion (emotional shock may cause the blood pressure to fall,
while rage may cause the blood pressure to rise).

312. **D** It has been said that emotional shock may cause the blood pressure to
fall (A). High blood pressure may be caused by narrowing of the arteries
(C). Alternatively, as the pressure of blood is increased, the arteries may
become thickened and narrowed (B). From this it can be seen that
hypertension may be either a symptom of disease or a cause of disease
(D).

313. **A** The most common cause of hypertension is vasoconstriction (narrowing
of the blood vessels). Think of the water tap again. If the pipes become
'furred' and narrowed, greater pressure is needed to push the water
through.

314. **A** We have seen how many factors work together to maintain normal blood
pressure. One of these factors is the state of the small blood vessels in
the skin. These vessels react to heat and cold in order to maintain normal
body temperature. Heat causes the vessels to dilate, which lowers the
blood pressure (B and D). Cold causes the vessels to contract, which
increases the pressure of blood (A). A sudden fright (C) produces a
state of shock and the blood pressure falls.

315. **B** Another factor which influences the blood pressure is the force with which the heart beats. The force must be sufficiently strong for oxygenated blood to reach all parts of the body. If you have ever overslept in the morning, you may have jumped out of bed immediately on waking. This action often has the effect of making you feel faint and giddy. This is because your brain was momentarily deprived of oxygen because the heart had to beat with greater force to push the blood upwards. This explains why, if a person receives a shock (lowering of the blood pressure) he should be encouraged to sit or lie down.

316. **D** Often hypertension is present for several years before producing symptoms. Gradually the blood vessels and heart show strain from the effects of the increased pressure. Headache is a common symptom and is often described by the patient as 'feeling like a weight on top of the head'. The headache is often accompanied by giddiness. The increased pressure may cause small blood vessels to rupture. This often occurs in the nose (epistaxis). The loss of blood can be severe and may result in a temporary lowering of the raised blood pressure. When a person has repeated episodes of bleeding from the nose, hypertension should always be considered as a possible cause.

317. **D** Hypertension may occur as a result of disease (e.g. nephritis).
318. **D** Alternatively, it may occur for no apparent reason and may cause disease
319. **A** due to the increased pressure. Hypertension for which no cause can be found is usually described as being either *essential* (also called benign essential), or *malignant*. Essential hypertension normally runs a slow course and it may be many years before the effects are apparent. Eventually the increased pressure will have varied and serious effects, which may include cerebral haemorrhage, heart failure and renal failure.

In contrast, malignant hypertension produces more severe symptoms in a shorter length of time, resulting in a rapid onset of complications, and the patient usually dies within a few years of the onset of symptoms, from a rapidly progressive uraemia.

There is no evidence that hypertension is a hereditary condition, although there is often a familial tendency to it.

320. **D** Blood leaves the left ventricle to travel via the aorta to the arteries. If the pressure of blood in the arteries is increased, the ventricle must work harder and this will cause it to enlarge and eventually fail to be effective in its function.

This added strain will eventually cause the right side of the heart to fail, due to back pressure in the left atrium causing congestion of the lungs.

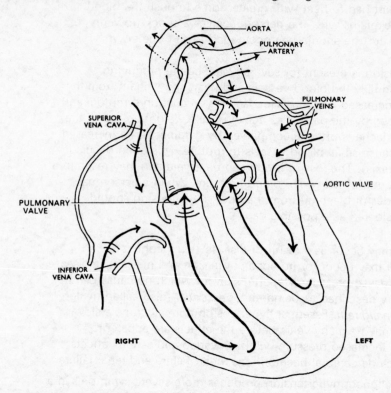

321. **D** Angina pectoris is a term used to describe severe but temporary cardiac
322. **A** pain. It commonly occurs as a result of exertion.
323. **A** The most common cause of angina is arteriosclerosis (321D). The
324. **D** sclerotic arteries are narrowed, which means that less blood is able to pass through them. This results in a reduction of the blood supply to the myocardium (322A), a condition known as ischaemic heart disease (323A).

Because the arteries are narrowed but not completely blocked, the diminished blood supply to the myocardium is usually adequate when the body is at rest. However, when activity is increased all the tissues of the body need an increased blood supply. In order to increase the blood supply, the heart beats faster. This means that the heart muscle needs an increased blood supply, but the coronary arteries are too narrow for extra blood to pass through, consequently, the heart muscle does not receive sufficient oxygenated blood for its increased activity and pain is felt (324D).

325. **A** We have seen how hypertension causes enlargement of the heart (answer 320). If the heart is enlarged it requires a greater amount of oxygen in order to function properly. The larger the heart, the more oxygen is required. Increased activity will further increase the demand for oxygenated blood and eventually pain will be felt because the myocardium is not receiving sufficient oxygenated blood.

326. **D** There are 1000 microgrammes in a milligramme therefore 500 microgrammes = 0.5 milligramme.

327. **B** Glyceryl trinitrate is a tablet which is effective in relieving angina if allowed to dissolve slowly under the tongue (sublingually).

328. **D** We have seen how angina occurs because the blood supply to the
329. **C** myocardium is inadequate. Therefore the aim of treatment is to improve
330. **C** the blood supply to the myocardium. This can be achieved by dilating the narrowed coronary vessels. Glyceryl trinitrate is effective in relieving the pain of angina (329C) because it is a vasodilator. As the coronary arteries dilate, more blood is able to reach the myocardium (330C). It should be remembered that glyceryl trinitrate does not *cure* the underlying cause of the angina, but relieves the symptoms, therefore it is given when symptoms occur (328D).

331. **A** When a person is unconscious, the priority is to ensure that the airway is kept clear of obstruction. This is assisted by keeping the patient in the semiprone position. Once the patient is in a safe position, the pulse may be taken (D).

Mr Dowling was *unconscious* and mouth-to-mouth resuscitation (B) and external cardiac massage (C) would not be required unless his respiratory and or circulatory systems had stopped functioning.

332. **C** Having ensured Mr Dowling's immediate safety, the next priority was to send for help. As there is a telephone in the room this would be the obvious choice, providing it was in working order (remember it had fallen onto the floor). Banging on the floor would be a very unreliable way of seeking help in these circumstances (B). Having assured herself that help was coming, Mrs Dowling could open a window and replace the furniture (D and A).

333. **A** Hopefully, Mrs Dowling will have performed all the actions listed, but the absolute priority is to ensure that domestic appliances have been switched off (cooker, iron, etc.)' Otherwise a fire may result which would not only damage the maisonette but may endanger the lives of other people living in the building. It is true that if the front door or windows are left open (D and B) an intruder could enter the dwelling which would be distressing to the Dowlings but not as distressing as loss of life caused by fire.

You may argue that this question 'all depends on circumstances' because you have no idea what Mr Dowling was doing when he was taken ill. However, you must remember that Mrs Dowling was out of the house when her husband was taken ill, so she had no idea what he was doing previously.

334. **C** When assessing the needs of a patient admitted to hospital the nurse should consider the patient's personal preferences (A), state of mobility (B) and social history (D), but the priority must be the patient's physical condition.

335. **D** We know that Mrs Dowling is a trained nurse but we do not know if she is familiar with the routine of an intensive care unit (A). Even if she is familiar with the routine, we must remember that she is experiencing a severe emotional disturbance. Her husband is very seriously ill and she will be feeling bewildered and upset. Because of this she should be treated with exactly the same sympathy and understanding as any other distressed relative. Sadly it is all too common for nurses whose relatives receive hospital care to say: 'If only they would understand that I can't see this in a detached, professional manner—it's not another patient to me, it's my husband/mother/daughter'.

336. **A** We have seen how angina is caused by a reduced blood supply to the
337.   myocardium due to narrowing of the coronary arteries. If a branch of the
            coronary artery should become completely blocked by a thrombus (clot),
            no blood can pass beyond that point, and the part of myocardium it
            supplies will die through lack of oxygen and nourishment.

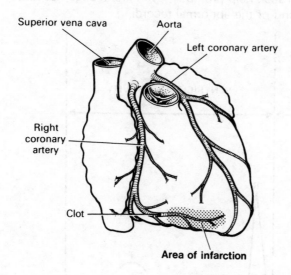

If a major branch of the coronary artery is blocked a large area of
myocardium will die and this may be incompatible with life of the
individual. Alternatively, if a minor vessel is blocked a comparatively
small area of myocardium will die.

This explains why some people die instantly and others make a full
recovery.

338. **A** When a nurse is first confronted with a cardiac monitor, she may find it rather alarming. It should be remembered though, that this is merely an aid to diagnosis and prompt detection of possible complications. The most important duty of the nurse is to learn to recognize normal sinus rhythm. If she is fully familiar with the *normal*, then she will recognize the abnormal and can seek help promptly, even if she does not fully understand the meaning of the abnormal recording.

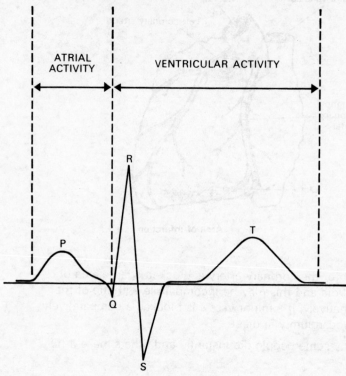

ATRIAL ACTIVITY   VENTRICULAR ACTIVITY

NORMAL SINUS RHYTHM

339. **D** The cardiac monitor is a mechanical device and like all machines it can develop faults. There may be an electrical fault or the leads may have become detached.

Look at the patient first, if he is a good, healthy colour, sitting up and chatting cheerfully, you can tell Sister this when reporting that the tracing is irregular. Alternatively, if the patient is collapsed or cyanotic you must seek help *immediately*.

340. **B** Whenever a patient dies, the heart stops beating and the circulation of blood ceases.

The term 'cardiac arrest' implies an emergency situation when there is a sudden cessation of the circulation in a patient who was not expected to die at that time. Age is not a vital criterion in determining cardiac arrest (C and D). The real criterion is the suddenness of the event.

341. **B** When a clot forms in a blood vessel it is known as a thrombus. If a piece of this clot breaks away and travels in the circulation it is known as an embolus.

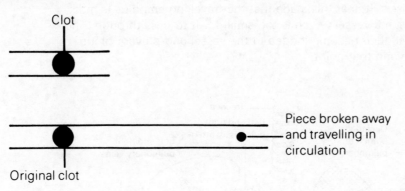

The embolus will continue to travel in the circulation until it reaches a vessel which is too small for it to pass through. The embolus will then become lodged in this vessel and no blood will be able to pass beyond it.

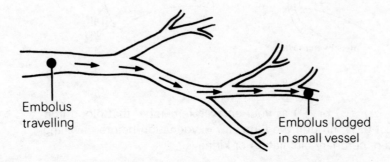

Blood from the veins returns to the right side of the heart and so the embolus would travel in this direction. Because the blood is returning to the heart, the veins are gradually joining to form larger vessels and the embolus will probably pass through without difficulty.

The next stage in the process of circulation is for the blood to pass from
the right ventricle to the lungs for oxygenation. As the pulmonary artery
enters the lung it gradually divides and subdivides into smaller and
smaller vessels. It is at this stage that the travelling embolus is most
likely to reach a vessel which is too small for it to pass through. The
embolus will then become lodged in the vessel and prevent blood
passing beyond that point.

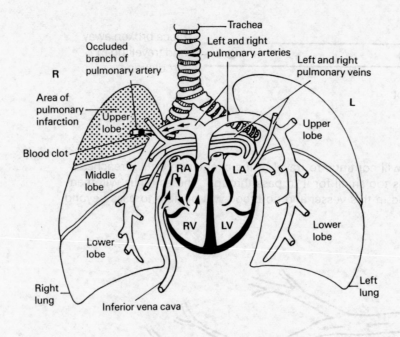

If you chose (A), (C) or (D) as your answer, remember that blood from
the veins must pass through the lungs for oxygenation before travelling
on to the brain, coronary circulation or kidneys.

342. **D** The choice of drugs for a patient's treatment depends on the doctor. However, nurses sometimes find it confusing when they are confronted with a patient who is being treated with anticoagulants for a deep vein thrombosis and yet another patient who has had a coronary thrombosis is not receiving anticoagulant therapy. This is because anticoagulants are generally considered to be more effective in the treatment of venous thrombi than arterial thrombi. It should be stressed though, that this is a general principle and there will be variations in treatment because the doctor assesses each patient individually when prescribing treatment. It is true that patients with a history of hypertension have a greater tendency to cerebro vascular accidents (B) but anticoagulants are unlikely to be used in preventive therapy.

343. **A**   To answer these questions it is necessary to understand something about
344. **A**   the clotting of blood. Our blood contains platelets and a variety of chemical substances in the plasma which are necessary for the formation of a clot. One of these substances is called prothrombin. Anticoagulant drugs destroy prothrombin and so prolong the clotting time, which should prevent further clots from forming. From this it can be seen that a clot which has already formed will not be affected by giving anticoagulant drugs.

345. **C**   We have seen how anticoagulant drugs act by delaying the clotting time
346. **D**   of the blood. However, it is important to ensure that the clotting time is not too slow, otherwise the patient is likely to bleed. This may be noticed first by blood in the urine (haematuria) or severe bruising of the skin.

   Haemophilia (345D) is a condition associated with bleeding. It is a hereditary condition, not associated with lack of prothrombin, but a lack of Factor 8 in the blood. (Factor 8 is a different chemical substance from prothrombin.)

347. **C**   In a normal healthy person the blood clotting time is kept at approximately the same level day and night. Anticoagulant drugs delay the clotting time but the aim should be to keep the blood at a constant level. This is achieved partly by giving the drug at the same time/times each day and partly by frequent regular blood estimations of the patient's prothrombin index.

   If the drug is given at erratic times, the blood levels of prothrombin will become erratic which could result in a misleading result to the blood test.

348. **D** In the initial stages of treatment, the aim is to reduce the clotting time of the blood as quickly as possible. Heparin has a more rapid effect than warfarin, which usually makes it the drug of choice at the onset of treatment. However, it has the disadvantage that it must be given by injection. Warfarin can be given orally but is slower to take effect. For this reason, many doctors prefer to give a combination of heparin and warfarin at the onset of treatment and discontinue the heparin when there has been a sufficient time lapse for the warfarin to become effective.

349. **D** Congestive cardiac failure is a term used when the right side of the heart
350. **A** fails to function properly. The right side of the heart is responsible for collecting deoxygenated blood from the body and passing it to the lungs for oxygenation. If the heart fails in this function, blood will not be sufficiently oxygenated and the patient will become dyspnoeic (breathless) and cyanosed. In addition, because blood is not passing effectively to the lungs it will collect in the right ventricle and atrium, causing 'overloading' of the venous system. Eventually severe congestion of the venous system will occur and this will result in oedema.

Acute chest pain (A and B) is relatively uncommon with cardiac failure. *Tachy*cardia (A and C) is usually present as the heart tries to compensate for the reduced oxygen content of the blood. If only the left side of the heart fails (B) this is known as left ventricular failure.

351. **C** Because the patient is dyspnoeic he should be nursed in the upright position. Lying the patient down (A, B and D) will increase the degree of dyspnoea.

352. **B** The diet for any person who is seriously ill should be light and easily digestible. This is particularly relevant to patients with congestive cardiac failure, partly because dyspnoea makes it difficult to eat (you will know this if you have ever had a severe chest infection) and partly to avoid overloading the digestive system.

353. **A** We have seen how severe congestion of the venous system gradually affects all parts of the body. The kidneys become congested and are unable to excrete salt properly, which is therefore retained in the body. Salt attracts water, so if salt is retained the degree of oedema will increase.

354. **D** Bacon (A), sausage (B) and haddock (C) all have a high salt content and would not be suitable for a salt-restricted diet. Eggs do not have a high salt content. The fact that the egg is fried will not affect the salt content (although it may not be so digestible). Salt-restricted diets can be very tedious and flavourless for some patients and nurses should try to offer suitable foods in a variety of ways. The routine 'boiled egg' for breakfast each day can become very monotonous particularly if the patient normally enjoys a liberal helping of condiments with an egg!

355. **C** Most nurses are familiar with the knowledge that digoxin 'slows and strengthens' the heart beat—but how does this happen?

Digoxin depresses the conducting tissues in the heart and this reduces the number of impulses which reach the ventricles. This results in a slowing of the heart rate and because the rate is slower, the beats are stronger and more efficient.

346. **C** There are 1000 microgrammes in a milligramme.

Therefore 250 microgrammes = 250/1000 milligramme.

= 0.25 milligramme.

357. **D** We have seen how digoxin slows the heart rate. Obviously it is important to ensure that the rate does not become too slow and this is why it is important for nurses to take the pulse before giving the drug. If the pulse rate is below 60, the drug is usually omitted. However, it is very important for the nurse to notify the person in charge of the ward and he/she will normally seek advice from the doctor. This is because, if the heart beat is very weak, the beats may not all be felt at the radial pulse. Consequently, the actual heart rate may be much faster than is detected by taking the pulse.

It is not sufficient to make a written note on the patient's treatment sheet as this may not be discovered until the next time drugs are due to be given.

358. **D** Frusemide is a diuretic. It is important to maintain a fluid balance chart in order to assess the patient's response to treatment with this drug.

359. **B** The purpose of giving a diuretic is to reduce oedema by increasing the patient's urinary output. If the drug is given early in the morning it should have had its maximum effect before the patient goes to sleep at night.

360. **C** Some diuretics (and frusemide is notable for this) increase the excretion of potassium from the kidneys. This potassium must be replaced and tablets of Slow K are commonly used for this. (Slow = slow release, K = chemical symbol for potassium). When oral potassium is given it is usually of the slow release type, otherwise it will simply be excreted again.

361. **D** All of the options will need attention but the priority is to relieve the dyspnoea by sitting the patient up. This should be done despite the fact that the sacral skin is red (B). Pressure should be relieved by moving the patient frequently.

362. **A** The three main causes of pressure sores are: unrelieved pressure, friction and moisture. Other factors which influence a person's susceptibility to pressure sores include lessened vitality and malnutrition (either overweight or underweight). Certain patients are more prone to pressure sores than others, especially those who are unconscious, paralysed, incontinent or oedematous. In addition, certain debilitating diseases increase a person's liability to develop pressure sores (e.g. diabetes and cancer).

From this it can be seen that all of the patients listed are at risk as they each come into one of the categories above, but the patient who is at *greatest* risk comes into more than one of the categories listed (bed rest + immobility + debilitating illness).

363. **C**   Different hospitals will have different types of fluid balance charts.
364. **C**
365. **B**

EXAMPLES

TIME	IN			OUT			COMMENTS
	Oral	I.V.	Blood	Urine	Vomit	Fistula	
Totals							

TIME	IN						OUT			COMMENTS
	ORAL		I.V.		BLOOD					
	Offered	Taken	Erected	Absorbed	Erected	Absorbed	Urine	Vomit	Fistula	
Totals										

Whichever type of chart is used, the principle is the same. *All* fluid intake and output should be recorded. The nurse should be diligent about this and record what is actually taken by the patient—patients have been known to use their drinking water for watering plants or refreshing their visitors!

Strict attention is also needed for accurate completion of the 'output' column. If a patient is incontinent, the nurse should be able to estimate the volume of fluid and write this on the chart with 'approximately' or 'estimated' beside it. It is *not* sufficient to write 'P.U.' or '+' or 'wet bed' as this gives no indication of the amount and 'P.U.' could mean anything from 50 ml to 500 ml.

366. **D** We have seen why oedema is a common symptom of congestive cardiac failure. Oedema is an excess of fluid in the tissues. This retention of fluid causes an increase in the patient's weight. Diuretic drugs are given to increase the urinary output and so relieve oedema. This should be evident by a corresponding loss of weight.

A nurse should observe her patients at meal times and notice if they are taking sufficient nourishment (A and B).

367. **A** Excess fluid may also collect in different cavities of the body. When it
368. **C** collects in the peritoneal cavity it is known as ascites. If the fluid collects
369. **A** in the pleural cavity it is known as hydrothorax.

Note.   When the term hydrothorax is used, it refers to fluid in the pleural cavity which has *not* occurred as a result of inflammation. When fluid is present in the pleural cavity as a result of inflammation (e.g. with pneumonia) it is known as pleural effusion.

370. **B** When a patient has ascites, the fluid in the peritoneal cavity causes the abdomen to be grossly distended. The fluid can be removed by inserting a cannula and allowing the fluid to drain slowly. The procedure is normally performed on the ward, under local anaesthetic. It is important that the patient's skin is clean (C and D), to avoid introducing infection. However, the most important duty of the nurse is to ensure that the bladder is empty, as a full bladder rises into the abdominal cavity and may be punctured accidentally when the trocar and cannula are introduced into the abdominal wall.

371. **B** The chest drain is inserted into the patient's pleural cavity. This drain is attached to the longer of the two tubes in the drainage bottle. The distal end of this tube *must* be immersed under the fluid in the drainage bottle. This is essential to prevent air being taken into the pleural cavity on inspiration. If you selected (A) as your answer to this question, think again—while it is vitally important to ensure that the chest drain is attached to the longer tube, this would be without purpose unless the distal end of the tube was immersed under fluid.

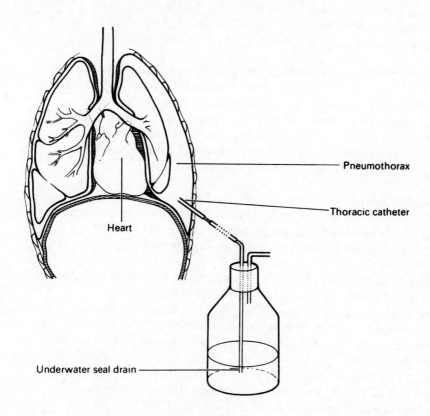

Pneumothorax

Thoracic catheter

Heart

Underwater seal drain

372. **D** This form of drainage is assisted by gravity. The bottle may have to be moved during nursing procedures (C)—for example, when moving the patient from his bed to a chair. However, it is very important that the bottle is not raised above the level of the lungs unless a clamp has been applied, as this will reverse the direction of the pull of gravity. Not only will drainage from the pleural cavity be prevented, but there is also a very grave risk of fluid from the bottle being sucked into the pleural cavity.

373. **C** We have seen that the distal end of the tube is immersed under fluid to prevent air being drawn into the pleural cavity. If the bottle is accidentally broken the fluid will be spilt and the end of the tube will be exposed. The nurse must apply a clamp to the tube as quickly as possible to prevent air being drawn into the pleural cavity. She must also be very careful to remember to remove the clamp once the drainage tube has been re-connected to a fresh drainage bottle. While it is important to protect the end of the tube from further contamination (D), the immediate priority is to prevent air entering the pleural cavity. Having dealt with these priorities the nurse should prevent further accident by taking appropriate action with the spilt fluid and broken glass (A and B).

374. **A** We have seen that it is very important to prevent air entering the pleural cavity. For this reason it is essential that the wound is sealed with an air-tight dressing immediately the drain is removed. (Collodian is a substance commonly used for this purpose.) Breathing exercises should be encouraged (D) and the patient's pulse and respiration rate should be recorded (B). Haemorrhage from the wound would not be expected following removal of this type of drainage tube (C).

375. **B** The notification of the family practitioner takes priority over the other three. If Mr Dowling was to become ill again shortly after his discharge, the doctor would be called and therefore it is essential that he has 'up to date' information of Mr Dowling's condition and treatment.

376. **D** Most hospitals encourage patients to be taken home from hospital by a relative or friend whenever possible. It is important for nurses to understand that each patient must be treated as an individual and consideration must be made of their social and domestic history as well as their physical condition. Mr Dowling lives in a maisonette with a long flight of steps leading to the door. Having recently been very seriously ill with heart failure he will need a great deal of assistance. The hospital car service will not be able to meet this need and for this reason he should be taken home by ambulance. A driver and attendant will then be available to help him with the stairs. If Mr Dowling had lived in a ground floor flat with easy access to the road, it would probably have been quite satisfactory for a member of his family to drive him home from hospital.

377. **C** Not all patients are fortunate enough to have a devoted family waiting for them, but it is important that there is someone available to receive them on discharge from hospital. If there are no relatives, an arrangement can usually be made with a neighbour. Failing this, the social worker may be able to make arrangements for someone to be available. This again shows the importance of knowing your patients and their domestic history. There is really no excuse for a patient being sent home from hospital to a cold, empty house, promptly having to start airing the bed and then shopping for essentials such as bread, butter and milk.

378. **C** Congestive cardiac failure is the term used to describe failure of the right side of the heart. This frequently develops following left ventricular failure (D) but may occur first in certain cases of chronic chest disease.

Congestive cardiac failure does not just 'happen' without an underlying cause. The causes of cardiac failure are many and very varied. Any condition which places strain on the heart is likely to result in cardiac failure. If the underlying cause can be cured (e.g. thyrotoxicosis) the patient's prognosis is more hopeful. Sadly, the majority of patients have an underlying heart condition which cannot be cured and the prognosis is very poor and relapses are frequent (C).

A few weeks after discharge Mr Dowling suffered a further myocardial infarction and died instantly. This was because a portion of his myocardium had died at the time of his original infarct, therefore the remaining heart muscle had to work harder to compensate. Eventually the extra strain caused the heart to cease functioning.

Chronic bronchitis

The following questions (379–425) are based on the case history below. They are all of the multiple choice type. Read each question and from the possible answers select the ONE which you think is correct.

Mr Campbell, aged 72 years has been admitted in a breathless and cyanotic state to an acute medical ward.

The patient is a bachelor who lives alone in a first floor rented flat. He is a cheerful man and has tried to maintain his independence as much as possible. His niece visits him about once a month and a good neighbour keeps a friendly eye on him.

Until his retirement at the age of sixty-five, Mr Campbell worked in the weights and measures department of a large bakery. For the past 12 years he has had 'chest trouble'. Originally this affected him only in the winter months but now he has a cough all the year round.

He has been admitted to hospital several times during the past few years with acute exacerbation of his chronic bronchitis. He is uncertain regarding dates of admission but states that they have become more frequent.

379. On admission to the ward, Mr Campbell was put into bed. Which of the following positions would be most suitable?
   A. Semi-recumbent
   B. Upright
   C. Recumbent
   D. Semi-prone.

379.

380. The doctor ordered that oxygen be given to Mr Campbell because of his cyanotic state. This would be given:
   A. At prescribed intervals on high concentration
   B. Continuously on low concentration
   C. Continuously on high concentration
   D. When necessary.

380.

381. All of the following are important in the administration of oxygen, but which should take priority?
   A. Check that the oxygen is given at the required concentration
   B. Identify the oxygen point or cylinder
   C. Use the appropriate mask or catheter
   D. Check that a humidifier is attached to the oxygen point.

381.

382. Which of the following is a danger associated with the administration of oxygen?
    A. Over-oxygenation of the surrounding atmosphere
    B. Dehydration of the patient
    C. Fire and explosion
    D. Rise in body temperature.

382.

383. Why is it necessary to use a humidifier when administering oxygen?
    A. To prevent dehydration
    B. To supplement the fluid intake
    C. To prevent halitosis
    D. To prevent irritation to the respiratory passages.

383.

As a young man, Mr Campbell was a heavy weekend drinker but now he only drinks socially. He began smoking when he was fifteen and for many years smoked 40 cigarettes a day. He says he now smokes only two or three cigarettes a day but this is doubtful.

On examination by the doctor, he presented a typical clinical picture of a person suffering from chronic bronchitis with the complication of emphysema.

384. Cigarette smoking aggravates the condition of chronic bronchitis. It can also cause:
    A. Bronchial carcinoma
    B. Coronary artery disease
    C. Visual disturbances
    D. All of the above.

384.

385. Chronic bronchitis is more common in:
    A. The adolescent
    B. The young child
    C. Middle-aged men
    D. Middle-aged women.

385.

386. Chronic bronchitis is associated with those who live in a climate which is:
    A. Warm and dry
    B. Cold and dry
    C. Cold and damp
    D. Warm and damp.

386.

387. Mr Campbell's bronchitis was aggravated by a:
   A. Poor diet
   B. Bad posture
   C. Obesity
   D. Dusty atmosphere.

387.

388. On looking at Mr Campbell's chest it was observed to be barrel shaped. This is due to:
   A. Increased residual air in the lungs
   B. Bad posture
   C. Enlargement of the diaphragm
   D. Continuous coughing.

388.

389. Mr Campbell showed signs of cyanosis. The cause of this is that the blood in the capillaries:
   A. Is increased
   B. Is decreased
   C. Lacks carbon dioxide
   D. Lacks oxygen.

389.

390. Dyspnoea was another of Mr Campbell's symptoms. This term means that breathing is:
   A. Laboured
   B. Rapid
   C. Shallow
   D. Noisy.

390.

391. All of the following signs were present on examination except one. Which one?
   A. Cyanosis
   B. Circumoral pallor
   C. Flared nostrils
   D. Pursed lips.

391.

392. Mr Campbell's cough was very troublesome and productive, and his sputum was:
   A. Thin and watery
   B. Blood stained
   C. Thick and white with black particles
   D. Thick, tenacious, yellow or green.

392.

393. Which of the following would be prescribed for his cough?
   A. Antibiotic
   B. Expectorant cough mixture
   C. Sedative cough mixture
   D. Broncho-dilator.

393.

394. Aminophylline was also prescribed. This is:
    A. An antibiotic
    B. A sedative
    C. A broncho-dilator
    D. An analgesic.

394.

395. During the acute stage of Mr Campbell's illness, aminophylline was given:
    A. Intravenously
    B. Intramuscularly
    C. Orally
    D. By inhalation.

395.

396. This drug, in the form of phyllocontin, 225 mg, is given orally, but must be:
    A. Swallowed whole
    B. Crushed
    C. Given sublingually
    D. Chewed.

396.

397. When the acute stage of the illness was over, the doctor prescribed aminophylline, 225 mg be given at night. Which of the following would be the most likely route?
    A. Orally
    B. Intramuscularly
    C. Intravenously
    D. Rectally.

397.

398. In addition, an antibiotic—amoxycillin 250 mg—was prescribed three times a day for:
    A. 10 days
    B. 1 month
    C. 3 months
    D. 6 months.

398.

At the beginning of his treatment, the physiotherapist was asked to visit Mr Campbell.

399. In the treatment of chronic bronchitis, the role of the physiotherapist is to:
    A. Give early ambulation
    B. Give leg exercises
    C. Give breathing exercises
    D. Check blood gases.

399.

400. The physiotherapist encouraged Mr Campbell to: 400.
    A. Use his diaphragm correctly
    B. To take short, shallow breaths
    C. Make use of his abdominal muscles
    D. Mouth breathe.

401. The physiotherapist instructed Mr Campbell in the use of an intermittent   401.
    positive pressure breathing ventilator. This apparatus may be used to:
    A. Administer drugs directly to the airway
    B. Improve aeration of the alveoli
    C. Aid the removal of secretions
    D. All of the above.

402. Mr Campbell had emphysema. This term describes: 402.
    A. Dilatation of the alveoli
    B. Thickening of the pleura
    C. Collapse of the lung
    D. Haemothorax.

403. Rupture of the alveoli may occur resulting in: 403.
    A. Bullae appearing on the lung surface
    B. Haematemesis
    C. Haemoptysis
    D. Fibrosis of lung.

404. As the lungs become less elastic there is an increase in: 404.
    A. Residual air
    B. Maximum breathing capacity
    C. Vital capacity
    D. Forced respiratory volume.

Mr Campbell was in hospital for 3 weeks. Initially on complete bed rest. This was followed by a gradual increase in activity in preparation for his return home.

---

405. The position Mr Campbell will assume in bed to ease his respiratory   405.
    difficulties can be achieved by the use of:
    A. A knee pillow
    B. A back rest and pillows
    C. A 'monkey pole'
    D. Sand bags.

406. Mr Campbell was bed bathed once a day. The main reason for this was to:
    A. Prevent pressure sores
    B. Allow the skin to function properly
    C. Reduce temperature
    D. Stop perspiration.

406.

407. When having a bed bath Mr Campbell was:
    A. Placed in the recumbent position
    B. Allowed to sit up in bed
    C. Allowed to wash himself
    D. Tepid sponged.

407.

408. Which of the following is it most important to observe during Mr Campbell's bed bath?
    A. Pressure areas
    B. Finger and toenails
    C. Respirations
    D. Texture of skin.

408.

409. Pressure area care was carried out:
    A. 4-hourly
    B. Daily
    C. When necessary
    D. After each meal time.

409.

410. Which of the following appliances would do most to relieve Mr Campbell's discomfort?
    A. A sheepskin
    B. Heel pads
    C. Overbed table and pillow
    D. Bed cage.

410.

411. How often would it be necessary for the nurse to inspect his mouth and carry out oral hygiene?
    A. 2-hourly
    B. 4-hourly
    C. Twice daily
    D. Daily

411.

412. Oral hygiene is essential to prevent:
    A. Infection
    B. Dehydration
    C. Herpes simplex
    D. Salivary duct calculi.

412.

413. Which of the following is important in maintaining oral hygiene?
    A. Adequate diet
    B. Adequate oral fluid intake
    C. Humidified oxygen
    D. Oral medication.

413.

414. Nutritional needs are important. Mr Campbell will benefit from:
    A. A high carbohydrate diet
    B. A diet low in roughage
    C. A salt-free diet
    D. A diet rich in protein.

414.

415. Meals should be served:
    A. When the patient feels hungry
    B. In small, easily digested amounts
    C. In semi-solid form
    D. In liquid form, e.g. Complan.

415.

416. It is essential that Mr Campbell has sufficient rest. This is important because it will reduce:
    A. His anxiety
    B. His vital capacity
    C. The oxygen demands of his body
    D. His weight.

416.

417. In order to ensure that Mr Campbell does not get too tired, the nurse should:
    A. Limit the number of his visitors
    B. Restrict his use of the radio
    C. Not allow him to feed himself
    D. Give a cough sedative.

417.

As Mr Campbell's condition improved, more activity was introduced into his day.

---

418. The increase in Mr Campbell's activity was based upon his:
    A. Nutritional intake
    B. Respiratory capabilities
    C. Pulse rate
    D. Temperature.

418.

419. During this increased activity it is particularly important to observe that:
    A. Diet is adequate
    B. Mobility is not tiring
    C. Bowel function is normal
    D. Temperature is normal.

419.

420. Due to his emphysema, Mr Campbell's tolerance to activity was decreased: 420.
    A. In the morning
    B. In the afternoon
    C. In the evening
    D. After meals.

During the next two weeks, Mr Campbell continued to make good progress. Preparations were made for his discharge home. He was taught various aspects of self-care in the hope of delaying the progression of his disease. He was advised to avoid activities which would produce excessive dyspnoea or lead to the recurrence of infection.

421. Which of the following would take priority in preventing breathlessness?   421.
    A. Breathing in a slow and relaxed manner
    B. Avoiding emotional stress
    C. Losing weight
    D. Adjusting his activities according to his fatigue pattern.

422. To prevent bronchial infections he was advised to: 422.
    A. Have rest periods before and after meals
    B. Take broncho-dilators as prescribed
    C. Practise pursed-lip breathing
    D. Avoid crowded places.

423. He was advised to develop good nutritional habits to prevent: 423.
    A. Infection
    B. Obesity
    C. Dyspnoea
    D. Cough.

424. To avoid exposure to respiratory irritants it is essential to: 424.
    A. Stop smoking
    B. Avoid extremely cold weather
    C. Avoid dusty atmospheres
    D. All of above.

425. It was arranged for Mr Campbell to have the services of one of the following   425.
    when he got home. Which one would be most beneficial?
    A. Meals on wheels
    B. Help the aged
    C. Home help
    D. District nurse.

Chronic bronchitis answers and explanations
(Questions 379 to 425)

379. **B** The upright position is used where there is respiratory embarrassment. This position makes expansion of the lungs easier for Mr Campbell. His back must be well supported with pillows and a back rest.

     The other positions would restrict breathing as the abdominal organs would tend to cause upward pressure on the diaphragm.

380. **B** The oxygen would be administered in a continuous low concentration using a face mask, e.g. Ventimask or nasal catheter.

     Patients with chronic bronchitis become anoxic with carbon dioxide retention. Carbon dioxide is normally the stimulus for the respiratory centre in the brain, but this stimulus is lost after a period of time as the centre becomes accustomed to the higher levels of carbon dioxide. The stimulus for respiration is now the low level of oxygen rather than the excess of carbon dioxide.

     Oxygen given at high concentration (A and C) or indiscriminately (D) may lead to higher than normal levels of oxygen in the blood. The respiratory centre would then have no stimulus and respiratory failure would result.

381. **B** All the options listed are important but the nurse must first check that the correct gas is being used. She should identify the oxygen point from bulk source or select the oxygen cylinder which is black with a white collar and the word 'oxygen' printed on it.

382. **C** All necessary precautions must be taken when oxygen is being administered to avoid the danger of fire and explosion. 'No smoking' signs are displayed in the vicinity, no oil or grease is used on oxygen apparatus, no sparking toys are allowed in a children's ward and antistatic materials must be used.

383. **D** When one breathes normally, the air entering the lungs is moistened. If oxygen is given without being humidified it will cause irritation of the respiratory passages and aggravate Mr Campbell's cough.

384. **D** Cigarette smoking can be a causative factor in (A) bronchial carcinoma, (B) coronary artery disease, and (C) visual disturbance where the optic nerve is damaged by the tobacco toxin.

385. **C** Chronic bronchitis is more common in men over the age of 40 although it can occur at any age in either sex.

386. **C** Those who live in a cold, damp climate, similar to that of Britain, are more at risk.

387. **D** Mr Campbell's condition was further aggravated by the fact that he had worked in a dust-laden atmosphere as a baker.

(A, B and C) can also be contributing factors.

388. **A** The typical 'barrel chest' of the chronic bronchitic results from air being trapped within the lungs as a result of their loss of elasticity.

There is anterio–posterior enlargement of the thorax and widening of the intercostal spaces. The ribs appear in the position of perpetual inspiration and the shoulders are raised.

389. **D** Cyanosis is the term used to describe the bluish discoloration of the skin resulting from a low concentration of oxygen in the blood and corresponding increase in the carbon dioxide level. It is usually indicative of a severe degree of respiratory disease.

390. **A** Dyspnoea means difficult, laboured and uncomfortable breathing (breathlessness). It is not always proportionate to the degree of respiratory embarrassment.

In patients with pulmonary dysfunction, breathing requires more effort, therefore more oxygen is required by the respiratory muscles. This creates a vicious circle which leads to fatigue and increased breathlessness.

In dyspnoea, respirations may be rapid, shallow and noisy (B, C and D) but not necessarily so.

391. **B** Circumoral pallor (a pale appearance of the skin around the mouth) occurs in fever and would not be present.

Cyanosis (A) is due to carbon dioxide retention and anoxia. Flared nostrils (C) occur in an attempt to increase the air intake. The lips are pursed (D) during expiration in an attempt to maintain the pressure in the air passages.

392. **D** The sputum is thick and tenacious. The yellow or green colour is due to the presence of infection. Anyone who has chronic bronchitis is advised to observe the colour of the sputum coughed up. As a rule the sputum is thick and white, and if the patient is a city dweller it is usually streaked with black particles (C).

The doctor should be consulted if the sputum changes in colour to yellow or green.

393. **B** It is necessary to encourage the removal of secretions from the lungs by giving the patient an expectorant cough mixture.

394. **C** The drug aminophylline is given to dilate the bronchi.

395. **A** During the acute stage of the illness, aminophylline is more effective if given slowly intravenously.

396. **A** Aminophylline (phyllocontin 225 mg) must be swallowed whole. Each tablet contains the drug in a unique controlled release system. If the tablet is chewed (D) or crushed (B) the slow release effect of the drug is lost.

397. **D** Aminophylline can be given rectally. The dose is usually one suppository inserted at night before retiring. This can be inserted by the patient himself. When given at this time it helps the patient to have a more peaceful night.

398. **A** Antibiotic therapy is usually prescribed for no longer than 10 days. Long-term use of an antibiotic reduces its effect. Because of frequent acute exacerbations of the condition it is necessary to prevent resistance to the antibiotic and this is achieved by giving it only when required and for a limited period.

399. **C** Physiotherapy is given to assist respiration. The therapist teaches the patient how to breathe more effectively, to use all the muscles of respiration and to make the cough more productive.

400. **A** With practice of breathing exercises, a better pattern of breathing should develop as the correct use of the diaphragm gives greater breathing control. The exercise should be carried out as follows:

    1.   The patient should sit upright in the bed or on a chair (preferably without arms) with his back well supported.

    2.   His fingers should be placed lightly on the front of his lower ribs, he should relax his shoulders and chest and breathe out as slowly as possible, feeling the lower ribs coming down and in towards the midline.

    3.   He should then breathe in and feel the slight expansion of his lower ribs under his fingers. This will give the sensation of breathing 'round the waist'.

401. **D** Intermittent positive pressure breathing is given by means of a pressure cycled ventilator which is driven by oxygen or compressed air. It can be delivered via a mouthpiece and is useful in the treatment of chest conditions. The addition of a broncho-dilating drug into the nebuliser of the ventilator enables the drug to be administered directly to the airway (A). This form of drug administration should not be given more than once every four hours.

    The ventilator produces more effective aeration of the alveoli (B) which results in aiding the removal of retained secretions (C).

402. **A** The alveoli become large and thin-walled. The lungs lose their elasticity.

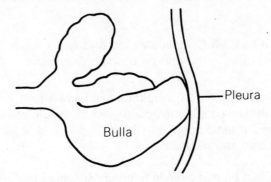

403. **A** Rupture of the alveoli results in large, watery blisters or bullae (singular—bulla) on the surface of the lung.

404. **A** As a result of distended alveoli and loss of elasticity in the lungs, expiration is more difficult, therefore residual air in the lungs is increased.

(B, C and D) are all reduced.

405. **B** To maintain an upright position and thus help in easing respiratory difficulties, a back rest and extra pillows are used. These must be placed in such a fashion to give good support with no gaps between the patient's back and the pillows, otherwise hollowing of the chest will result.

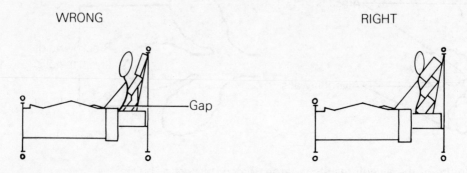

WRONG   RIGHT

—Gap

406. **B** Daily bathing will keep the skin clean and fresh and allow it to function properly.

407. **B** When having his bath in bed, Mr Campbell would find it much less distressing to be allowed to sit in the upright position during the procedure.

   If placed in the recumbent position (A) respiratory embarrassment would result. If allowed to wash himself (C) the added exertion would cause further respiratory distress. If tepid sponged (D) chilling would occur and leave Mr Campbell cold and miserable.

408. **C** General observations would be made while bathing Mr Campbell, but it is important to pay close attention to his respirations in order to detect any changes that may occur during the effort of being bathed. It may be necessary to allow short rest periods during the bathing to reduce the amount of oxygen required and prevent fatigue.

409. **A** Mr Campbell was encouraged to change his position in bed frequently, but not to overtax his energy. His pressure areas were inspected four-hourly and the necessary care was given.

410. **C** An overbed table with a pillow placed on it provides support for the patient's arms. This allows the use of the accessory muscles of respiration to assist in lifting the rib cage. This helps to relieve breathlessness.

   (A, B and C), while giving comfort, can assist in preventing pressure sores developing, and do nothing to improve breathing difficulties.

411. **A** Two-hourly care of the mouth is necessary. Patients with chronic bronchitis tend to mouth breathe, which causes dryness of the mouth. Oxygen therapy, even in low concentration, also causes the mouth to become dry.

412. **A** It is necessary to carry out oral hygiene regularly to prevent infection of the mouth developing. This infection can spread to the already diseased lungs.

413. **B** An adequate oral fluid intake will assist in keeping the mouth moist and clean.

414. **D** Mr Campbell will benefit from a diet rich in protein. Among its many functions, protein is essential to build and repair body tissue and to aid the body to resist disease.

   A diet rich in carbohydrate (A) would tend to increase Mr Campbell's weight which would aggravate his condition by making more demand on oxygen. A low roughage diet (B) would make him constipated.

415. **B** Meals should be served in small, attractive, easily digested amounts. The effort of eating, plus the digestion of food makes quite a demand on the oxygen available. The added effort of trying to cope with large meals soon exhausts the patient, with the result that loss of appetite can result from fear of causing further respiratory distress.

416. **C** Adequate rest will reduce the oxygen demands of the body. To force the body into unnecessary activity is not only distressing to the patient but is also dangerous as respiratory failure may result.

417. **A** Assured rest is assisted by limiting the number of visitors. Too many visitors are tiring for most patients. Patients who are dyspnoeic have the added strain of increased oxygen demand in an effort to make extra conversation.

418. **B** As Mr Campbell's condition improved, a more balanced form of rest and activity was introduced. His respiratory capabilities must be taken into account as more activity is undertaken. This increase in activity is also necessary to prevent other complications and boredom.

419. **B** Observations must be made during this increased activity to note if mobility is tiring. If oxygen demands by the body are too great then the form of activity must be altered to cope with the oxygen available.

   The other observations (A, C and D) should be made at all stages of his treatment.

420. **A** Tolerance to activity is usually decreased first thing in the morning. This is due to secretions gathering in the lungs during the night, which results from bad posture occurring while the patient is asleep (sliding down in the bed from the upright position to a more reclining position). This leads to a reduction in the capacity of the lungs with little or no reserve of oxygen for physical activity.

421. **D** While all could be of benefit to Mr Campbell, it is necessary for him to adjust his individual pattern of life to meet the demands of his body for oxygen.

422. **D** To reduce further attacks of bronchial infection he was advised to avoid overcrowded areas and contact with persons known to have colds or other infections.

423. **B** Obesity puts added strain on the heart and lungs which in turn increases dyspnoea. This can be avoided by eating regularly and taking a diet which is nutritional and easily digested.

424. **D** There are many respiratory irritants but those listed (A, B and C) can to some extent be prevented. Smoking must be discouraged and the dangers and hazards it causes to health should be pointed out. No one can compel the patient to stop smoking but he should be advised to reduce his intake to a minimum.

     Extremely cold weather may be avoided by staying indoors when necessary. If he has to go out, a scarf over nose and mouth warms the inspired air.

     Dusty atmospheres or fumes irritating to the respiratory passages should be avoided.

425. **C** It was arranged for a home help to be available five morning per week, Monday to Friday. She would attend to household chores, do light necessary shopping and prepare meals.